Emergence of Medicine from the "Dark Ages"

Edward R. Lang M.D.

Copyright © 2018 by Edward R. Lang M.D.

Library of Congress Control Number:		2018912799
ISBN:	Hardcover	978-1-9845-6245-6
	Softcover	978-1-9845-6244-9
	eBook	978-1-9845-6243-2

All rights reserved. No part of this book may be reproduced or transmitted in any form or by any means, electronic or mechanical, including photocopying, recording, or by any information storage and retrieval system, without permission in writing from the copyright owner.

The views expressed in this work are solely those of the author and do not necessarily reflect the views of the publisher, and the publisher hereby disclaims any responsibility for them.

Any people depicted in stock imagery provided by Getty Images are models, and such images are being used for illustrative purposes only.
Certain stock imagery © Getty Images.

Print information available on the last page.

Rev. date: 10/30/2018

To order additional copies of this book, contact:
Xlibris
1-888-795-4274
www.Xlibris.com
Orders@Xlibris.com

Contents

Introduction v

Chapter 1	Anesthesia	1
Chapter 2	Hygiene and Public Health	5
Chapter 3	Education	16
Chapter 4	Physiology	20
Chapter 5	Part 1: Dr. Cushing's War	26
	Part 2: Principles of Wound care and Outcome	30
Chapter 6	The End of the beginning	32
Chapter 7	Radiology: A great leap forward in medical diagnosis	36
Chapter 8	Immunology: the viral scourge	39
Chapter 9	Beyond Observation and Support: The Physician comes of Age	45
Chapter 10	Part 1: Pharmacology comes of age: Antibiotics and beyond	52
	Part 2	58
Chapter 11	Surgical surprises-encounters with unexpected pathology	61
Chapter 12	Part 1: Tuberculosis and the emergence of thoracic surgery	65
	Part 2: Dawn of cardiovascular surgery	70
Chapter 13	Part 1: Hospitals and training	73
	Part 2: Hospitals and Training	77
	Part 3	81

Chapter 14 Challenge of Protozoan and Fungal illness in mid twentieth century 84
Chapter 15 Nutritional essentials: The role of selectivity in health and disease... 87
Chapter 16 Part 1: Poisoning: Intentional and accidental 89
Part 2: Opioid crisis 91

Endnotes 95

Introduction

From the perspective of the twentieth century it is apparent that the majority of inhabitants of North America and Western Europe share the expectation of general good health. While some may achieve this goal through regular exercise and appropriate nutrition, many individuals rely upon modern scientific medical practice to ensure health maintenance. The physiologic basis for medical guidance and treatment has only been understood and become available to the public since the early decades of the twentieth century-a very short time indeed. One only need recall that during the early nineteenth century illness was commonly treated by "bleeding and purging" (often with disastrous results) by physicians who had little understanding of disease mechanism or viable treatment options.

Since the Renaissance and Reformation of the fifteenth and sixteenth centuries, advances in physical science had produced steam, electric power and the telegraph allowing rapid human communication at a distance by the 1860s. Unfortunately the majority of significant advances in medicine and public health were delayed until later in 19th century. In this volume it is our intention to describe and explore major contributions to human health which occurred in an explosive fashion between the American Civil War and the mid-20th century.

Appalling sanitary conditions typical for the period were described by Torvald in regard to the "barracks" Hospital of Scutari during the Crimean War Although highly motivated, intensive efforts made by Florence Nightingale and her dedicated staff to alleviate the continuous suffering of the wounded in this conflict were largely limited by absence of the "germ theory of disease". Sadly for the patients this knowledge lay a decade in the future. In 1853 shocking ignorance of sanitation and hygiene persisted from battlefield to treatment center for the majority of the wounded. Thus bacterial infection of injury was eventually guaranteed in almost all cases in which the body had been penetrated by a foreign object. If the missile or blade had not introduced microbial Invaders then surely the surgeons, nurses and others attending the patient did so. Contributing further to contamination of wounds was the extreme delay in removing the injured soldiers from the battlefield. In 1863, during the American Civil War, Jonathan Letterman,(Surgeon General of the Army of the Potomac) introduced a primitive ambulance service.[1] This effort provided limited psychological and spiritual assistance for the wounded even though overall morbidity and mortality were little diminished. Suffice it to acknowledge that essentially no advances of major significance in medical treatment had been made since the Revolutionary War while surgery was primarily limited to amputation of shattered limbs under primitive conditions.

Robert Denney's Illuminating volume" Civil War Medicine" aptly sets the stage for an understanding of the plight of soldiers and civilians prior to the late 19th century.[2] At that time survivors of childhood diseases lived to an average age of 55 years. "Operating methods were primitive and wholly unsanitary. Diarrhea and dysentery affected two-thirds of all troops during the first year of service. In spite of inadequate scientific understanding of the nature of disease a U.S. Sanitary Commission was formed which issued pamphlets on the use of latrines as well as personal hygiene. Further

---

1   Chapman, Carleton B. *Order out of Chaos*. New York: Carleton B. Chapman Science History Publications/USA,1992.

2   Denney, Robert. *Civil War Medicine: Care and Comfort Of the Wounded*. New York: Sterling Publishing Co., 1994.

impairment of health was produced by a diet limited in vitamins and protein. Even food which might initially have been considered nutritious was frequently permitted to spoil before becoming available to the troops". Denny notes that in 1861 the chief US medical officer was a veteran of the War of 1812. The Civil War began with a total of 98 medical personnel to support 16,000 regular Army troops. Nurses were essentially untrained American women such as Louisa May Alcott who volunteered to be of service to their country and its military.[3] The reader will appreciate that although <u>diagnosis</u> of certain conditions had improved, progress in treatment of many ailments had progressed very little even by the advent of WWI.

In June 1862 Jonathan Letterman became Medical Director of the Army of the Potomac. Trained at Jefferson Medical College he had been appointed assistant surgeon in the army in 1849. Disorganization of the army early in the Civil War was such that colonels of some state regiments refused to accept medical officers appointed to them by law--an economic conflict. Obviously wounding was only a portion of the army's medical problem. Letterman wrote "The deadly malarial poison....was now being fully manifested in the prevalence of malarial fevers of a typhoid type, diarrheas, and scurvy". Soldiers of the New Hampshire Volunteers arrived at Hilton Head Island in 1862 carrying the dreaded Yellow Fever from Key West.

Early in 1862 a report on improving health in the Northern Army of the Potomac described 247,000 cases of disease and injury. Included herein were 40,000 cases of diarrhea and dysentery, 10,000 cases of typhoid fever, along with more than 7500 infected with syphilis and gonorrhea.[4] A dramatic increase in intestinal infections occurred as the war progressed: Between 1861 and 1865 the mortality from typhoid fever had increased from 17% to 56% in the Union Army. It was truly a "Dark Age" from which Medicine emerged

---

3 Denney, Robert. *Civil War Medicine: Care and Comfort of the Wounded*. New York: Sterling Publishing Company,1994. pp.186-187

4 Denney, Robert. *Civil War Medicine: Care and Comfort of the Wounded*. New York :Sterling Publishing Company,1994.

during the ensuing century. Control of this problem was determined by extensive improvement in public health measures and the eventual development of antibiotics. Massie writes in "Castles of Steel" that of 34,000 casualties of the Gallipoli landings (1915) 14,000 were incapacitated by disease.[5]

---

[5] Massie, Robert K. *Castles of Steel*. 2003

CHAPTER 1

Anesthesia

Surely the greatest blessing for individuals subjected to wounding and invasive medical procedures during the 19th century was the introduction of anesthesia. In 1842 a Georgian, Crawford Long, administered ether to a man requiring an operation on his neck.[6] This new concept qualifies as one of the earliest medical "miracles". Several years later Dr. Morton provided ether anesthesia for a patient operated on at the Massachusetts General Hospital by Dr. Warren. In 1847 Sir James Simson introduced chloroform as an anesthetic at the Edinburgh Royal Infirmary. By 1853 Queen Victoria had been given chloroform anesthesia for childbirth.[7] As has been common with numerous therapeutic innovations, marked resistance to the introduction of anesthesia was encountered. Many physicians and laymen believed that suffering pain was truly "the will of God." While some practitioners denounced anesthesia as a dangerous and blasphemous novelty, most doctors cautiously accepted it as a mixed blessing that had to be used selectively. Opponents of surgery

---

6   Porter, Roy. *The Greatest Benefit to Mankind*. New York, London: Horton and Company,1997. p367

7   Porter, Roy. *The Greatest Benefit to Mankind*. New York, London: Horton and Company,1997. p367

performed under anesthesia openly pounced upon reports of death following the operation neglecting the fact that many patients died without the benefit of anesthesia. It is of paramount importance for the reader to appreciate the vast difference between the basic relief of pain and the safety and security of modern anesthesiology which is currently taken for granted. At the time of its introduction several things concerning the chemical and physiological nature of ether rapidly became apparent which were of consequence both to the patient and those attending in the operating theatre. Foremost was the inflammability of this compound that subjected all involved to the hazard of fire and explosion-especially if cautery was being used. In contrast to the benefit of pain relief during surgery was a formidable risk incurred by patients in the absence of monitoring of their vital signs- prior to the turn of the 20th century. In general no recording of the patient's pulse, respiration and blood pressure was made while under anesthesia during the last decade of the 19th century. Harvey Cushing, (father of American neurosurgery) while a medical student at Harvard, administered general anesthesia for the surgeons at the Massachusetts General Hospital who were unaware that the patient was barely alive.[8]

Dr. T G. Morton in "Hospital Reports" of the Pennsylvania Hospital clearly describes the detail of providing anesthesia for an amputation in 1865. "The gas is carried in a gutta–percha bag having a flexible tube and hard rubber mouthpiece. The patient takes full breaths. Total anesthesia is induced in 20-30 seconds".[9] An alternative to ether, e.g. nitrous oxide- had been discovered by Joseph Priestly in 1776 and was minutely examined by Sir Humphrey Davy in 1805. Its successful application in dental anesthesia was described in the Boston Medical and Surgical Journal. In this article H.J. Barnes M.D. purports to show that Nitrous Oxide ".. may be made useful

---

[8] Fulton, John Farquhar. *Harvey Cushing, a Biography*. Springfield: Charles Thomas, 1946.

[9] Morton, T.G. "Surgical Clinic by Dr. T.G. Morton". *Hospital Reports of the Pennsylvania Hospital*, Oct 12, 1865.

and practicable in place of ether, for painful examinations, short operations, and the adjustment of broken bones...". He further states that the gas.. "has been administered by them (Drs. Ball and Fitch) not less than 15,000 times".[10] Deaths from the ether drip methods were not infrequent and well-documented in Fulton's "Harvey Cushing"- eventually leading to the introduction of The Ether Chart. It is clear that death following surgical intervention at that time was poorly understood by all those involved in the surgical procedure.[11] One of Cushing's earliest contributions to scientific medicine was the introduction of a cuff for the measurement of blood pressure (during an operation) which he had observed while studying in Europe. Although deaths were decreased, the risk of general anesthesia remained high primarily related to the method of administration. One refinement of anesthetic technique was described by M.H. Rogers- pathologist to the Bristol, England Hospital for Sick Children in 1895. He notes that "all the unpleasant sensations experienced during the early stages of ether anesthesia may be avoided by giving a small amount of nitrous oxide first". He subsequently condemns the use of chloroform regarding which he states that "..patients not infrequently pass to a more or less dangerous stage with great and unexpected suddenness[12]. Van Hook of Chicago wrote in 1904 that giving a small amount of nitrous oxide prior to administration of ether allows a more pleasant experience for the patient and lowers the amount of ether required for anesthesia.[13] Initially anesthetic agents such as ether and chloroform were administered by dripping the liquid onto a porous mask applied to the patient's nose and mouth. The

---

10   Barnes, H.J. M.D. "Nitrous Oxide Gas" *Boston Medical and Surgical Journal*, 1874, pp. 511-513.

11   Fulton, John Farquhar. *Harvey Cushing, a Biography*. Springfield: Charles C. Thomas, 1946.

12   Rogers. Administration of Nitrous Oxide preliminary to Ether Anesthesia. *Medical and Surgical Reporter*, vol. 84, no.26, June 8,1895, p81

13   Van Hook, William M.D. "Apparatus for Nitrous Oxide –Ether Anesthesia" *Chicago Medical News*(1882-1905) June 18, 1904, pp. 84, 25.

concentrations of such compounds reaching the recipient's lungs and by extension entering the blood and brain were largely unknown and fluctuated widely. Inadequate pain relief or possible fatal overdoses were not unusual outcomes.

Endotracheal intubation for safe administration of gaseous anesthetics was not introduced until well after World War 1. Around 1913 Chevalier Jackson had developed an early form of bronchoscope and laryngoscope allowing for the first time accurate visualization of the channel through which an endotracheal tube could be passed. This eventually permitted the use of gas anesthesia with agents such as cyclopropane and elimination of the dangerous drip methods.

In 1871 Trendelenburg in Germany published a paper describing an elective tracheotomy designed to permit administration of general anesthesia. William McEwen (Scotland) reported on intubation via the mouth enabling respiration in a case of obstruction of the glottis(airway) due to pathologic swelling. By 1895 direct visualization of the larynx was demonstrated by Alfred Kirstein, the critical step in safe administration of general endotracheal anesthesia as practiced in the twentieth century. Prior to accurate placement of the tube into the trachea, laryngeal spasm, airway blockage as well as vomiting with aspiration of gastric contents had been life-threatening risks preceding the surgical anesthesia. Subsequent addition of an inflatable cuff to the tube markedly reduced the risk of aspiration of gastric contents into the lungs. However as recently as 1966 the author witnessed an anesthetic related death in a 12 year old boy whose esophagus rather than the trachea had been inadvertently intubated leading to asphyxiation. During the 1930's rapid and clearly safer methods of anesthetic induction were achieved through the use of short acting intravenous drugs such as thiopental (Pentothal) and muscle relaxants which facilitated intubation further reducing the risk of aspiration and airway obstruction. Carbon dioxide absorbers and oximetry to measure blood oxygen levels further increased safety by the decade of the sixties.

Chapter 2

Hygiene and Public Health

In a thorough documentation of the state of medicine and human health in America during and beyond the Civil War Chapman produced "Order out of Chaos" describing in detail the life and times of John Shaw Billings. As a young military surgeon Billings witnessed the bloodiest days in American history including the slaughter at Antietam and Gettysburg. Although little could be done at the time to ameliorate the situation, Billings was clearly aware that morbidity and mortality from disease was virtually equal to that of wounding in battle. Early in the war Billings served in Washington, DC as director of the Cliffburne hospital in Georgetown.[14] In 1862 he was transferred to the Philadelphia General Hospital. After exhausting service at both Chancellorsville and Gettysburg in 1863, he was given 30 days relief from duty. Following the war Billings became part of a team in the Surgeon General's office which wrote "the Medical and Surgical History of the War of the Rebellion".[15] This multiple volume tome appears to represent the first effort to

---

[14] Chapman, Carleton B. *"Order out of Chaos"*. Boston: Carleton B. Chapman,1992, p61.

[15] Chapman, Carleton B. *"Order Out of Chaos"*. Boston: Carleton B. Chapman, 1992. p78

comprehensively document large numbers of medical and surgical cases occurring during the war. The reader should understand that prior to this time much of medical reporting was simply anecdotal allowing little if any analysis which might improve future results. In 1875 Billings published "Report on the Hygiene of the United States Army" which espoused improved hospital construction with physical separation of the wards of different types of cases, better ventilation, and non- allowance of double deck beds. By 1874 he had become a member of the design team creating the new Johns Hopkins hospital in Baltimore. Subsequently he was appointed professor of Hygiene at the Medical school where he retained an appointment as Lecturer until 1904. Meanwhile working for the. US government, Billings began to compile what was eventually to become the National Library of Medicine. By 1885 he had amassed a collection of 85,663 volumes. Finally he produced "Index Catalogue of the Library of the Surgeon General's office", later known as "The Index Medicus".[16]

A major effort to bring a semblance of improved hygiene to the Union armies evolved through the efforts of the U.S. Sanitary commission formed in New York in 1861 through the efforts of Dr. Henry Bellows and representatives of ladies' relief societies. This organization was officially commissioned on June 9, 1861 by the secretary of war and President Lincoln.[17] Mary Ann Bickerdike of Galesburg, Ill. was appointed to inspect the Union "hospital" in Cairo (Ill.) Following is a report by Frederick Olmsted, a senior member of the commission. "The camps were located in poor areas with no provision for drainage.....latrines were just trenches about 30 feet long without pole or rail, the stench almost overpowering; the men's clothing was filthy and no attempt had been made to get them to a bathing facility". Contamination of the water supply in many camps produced widespread dysentery and frequent cases of typhoid fever. A

---

16   Chapman, Carleton B. *"Order out of Chaos"*. Boston: Carleton B. Chapman Science History Publications/USA, 1992, p.171

17   Denney, Robert. *Civil War Medicine: Care and Comfort of the Wounded*. New York: Sterling Publishing Company, Inc. p24, 37, 44.

Emergence of Medicine from the "Dark Ages"

surgeon described the conditions subsequent to the battle of Wilson's Creek, Missouri... "the flies were extremely troublesome ....maggots forming in the wounds in less than an hour after dressing them".[18] They were finally eliminated by sprinkling calomel over the wounded areas. Medication available for prescription at this time were limited to opioid narcotics, purgatives, emetics and plant extracts of dubious value. It follows that almost all improvement in healthcare depended on reducing bacterial contamination of food, water, clothing and bedding in conjunction with improved nutrition and personal hygiene of the patient. Major efforts in the enhancement and development of hospital care will be considered in a subsequent chapter.

In spite of limited scientific understanding of the etiology and pathogenesis of infectious disease efforts were undertaken to combat epidemic health crises in the 19th century. In England industrialization produced overwhelming overcrowding in the cities. The population of London rose from 800,000 in 1801 to 8,000,000 in 1901 with intense overcrowding and totally inadequate sanitary infrastructure. The "Poor Laws" provided for some structural shelter and rudimentary health care for the "dregs of society".[19] Removal of certain individuals from society at large probably served to reduce epidemic spread of disease although cause and effect were poorly understood. A major outbreak of Cholera in SoHo (London} apparently was enough to convince John Snow in 1854 that the disease was transmitted via contaminated drinking water. Measures taken to eliminate the polluted well dramatically reduced progression of the illness in the local population. The Public Health Act of 1875 required appointment of a medical official to every sanitary district in England. The squalor of living conditions produced a massive epidemic of Typhus. Between 1917 and 1921 about 25 million cases were reported.

---

18 Straubing, Harold. *In Hospital and Camp: The Civil War through the Eyes of its Doctors and Nurses*. Stackpole Books. 1993.

19 Porter, Roy. *The Greatest Benefit to Mankind*. New York, London: Horton and Company,1997.

Public Health progress in America lagged behind Britain related primarily to relative size and rural nature of the territory. In 1800 only 33 American towns had populations greater than 2500. Around mid-19th century Griscom (Health Inspector of New York City) believed that to follow the rules of hygiene was a "moral act and religious duty". Believing cholera's primary predisposing cause to be sin (intemperance, atheism, vice and greed) the hygienic gospel was preached".[20] As we have previously described, the American Civil War provided an additional stimulus to Public Health in the United States.

In his outstanding review of 20th century medicine,"The Youngest Science", Lewis Thomas, an immunologist and pathologist, allows us to glimpse the physician's role at the onset of the 20th century He bases this information on observations made while doing rounds in homes with his father, a family physician in Flushing, New York. Dr. Thomas insists that prior to World War 1 the doctor was primarily an interpreter and caretaker. [21] Although diagnostic identification of specific medical diseases had begun to evolve through the efforts of such giants as Sir William Osler (at Johns Hopkins) very little active treatment was available to the practitioner. Physicians primarily offered diagnosis, prognosis and emotional support to the patient and family while awaiting the eventual outcome of the illness. Although this period offered dramatic advances in surgical management of several common conditions i.e. appendicitis, breast cancer and hernia repair, the majority of non-surgical progress occurred in the field of hygiene and Public Health. Following years as a pathologist, Dr. Thomas had acquired little exposure to public health issues prior to appointment to the New York City Health Board in 1956.[22] This

---

20 Porter, Roy. *Greatest Benefit to Mankind*. New York, London: Horton and Company, 1992.

21 Thomas, Lewis. *Medicine: The Youngest Science*. New York: The Viking Press,1983, p.270

22 Thomas, Lewis. *Medicine: The Youngest Science*. New York: The Viking Press, 1983.

appears especially surprising since courses in hygiene and public health were being offered in some universities as early as 1916. During the latter half of the 19th century multiple epidemics of Cholera spread throughout Europe eventually reaching as a pandemic to North America. Such disasters could only be controlled by public health measures including quarantine. [23]

It seems self-evident to trace the onset of improved public health to the identification and description of the process of fermentation and putrefaction by Louis Pasteur whose seminal discovery occurred during the late 1860's in France in the face of intense resistance by that country's medical elite. Pasteur was able to unequivocally demonstrate the falsity of the age-held doctrine of "spontaneous generation". He showed that a sterile solution remains sterile for days or weeks as long as contaminating bacteria are not introduced from without into the original container.[24] In 1879 Pasteur showed that chickens could be immunized against Cholera. By 1881 he had shown conclusively that sheep and cows could be protected from anthrax by immunization. His ultimate triumph occurred in 1885 when his anti-rabies serum vaccine saved the lives of two boys bitten by mad dogs.[25] Based on Pasteur's revelations, Joseph Lister in Glasgow introduced the concept of antisepsis in surgery and treatment of wounds. During the 1870s Lister began to spray both the operating theatre and patients with carbolic acid which was bactericidal.[26] While such chemicals were commonly irritating to skin and other human tissue, the reduction in infection rate was dramatic. Of particular significance was Lister's ability to save injured limbs from the accepted treatment: amputation.

---

23 Porter, Roy. *The Greatest Benefit to Mankind*. New York, London: Horton and Company, 1997.

24 Porter, Roy. *The Greatest Benefit to Mankind*. New York, London: Horton and Company, 1997. pp431-5.

25 Porter, Roy. *The Greatest Benefit to Mankind*. New York, London: Horton and Company,1997, pp434-5.

26 Torvald, Jurgen. *The Century of The Surgeon*. New York :Pantheon Books Inc.,1956.

As had been the case with Pasteur, enormous resistance to this new technique was encountered from established surgeons. Prior to aseptic techniques, invasive surgical procedures which entered the chest, abdomen and brain almost uniformly led to infection and fatality. A recent documentary film provided by PBS emphasized the role of infection in the death of president James A. Garfield in 1881. Although the gunshots did not compromise vital organs, frequent probing and contamination of wounds by unwashed hands and instruments eventually led to overwhelming sepsis and death about 10 weeks after the shooting.

In 1882 Robert Koch presented his research to the Berlin Physiologic society which identified the Tubercle Bacillus as the cause of tuberculosis [27] a major infectious agent which produced extensive human morbidity and mortality. By 1883 Koch had also identified the bacillus which caused cholera and attributed transmission of the disease to polluted water. Following the identification of the anthrax bacillus (Pasteur) and the tubercle bacillus, a host of additional pathogenic organisms were described during the last decades of the 19th century by researchers in France and Germany. Among the most important of those identified were Salmonella Typhi (typhoid fever), Corynebacterium diphtheriae and clostridium tetani (tetanus or "'lockjaw").[28] Immunity could be conferred by injecting the serum of a person (or animal) previously infected into a non-immune individual. Many lives were saved during the early 20th century by vaccination against tetanus and typhoid. Childhood mortality was dramatically reduced by widespread diphtheria immunization. At this time further understanding of immunity and resistance to infection developed following the work of Metchnikoff, a Russian pathologist working at the Pasteur Institute. Around 1884 he identified cells which were microscopically seen to have engulfed or ingested bacteria in the blood

---

27 Porter, Roy. *The Greatest Benefit to Mankind*. New York, London: Horton and Company, 1997, pp 440-442.

28 Porter, Roy. *The Greatest Benefit to Mankind*. New York, London: Horton and Company, 1997, pp437-445.

and tissue of infected animals. He named these leukocytes (white blood cells) "phagocytes".[29] It was subsequently shown that phagocytic ingestion of bacteria was enhanced significantly by the presence of "immune" serum. Thus resistance to infection is determined by a cellular attack on invasive bacteria enhanced by chemical substances found in the blood serum of immunized individuals In contrast to the limited treatment available to *individual* patients, hygiene and preventive medicine played a major role in widely improving human health at the turn of the 20th century.

In 1879 a National Board of Health was developed. Supported by Theodore Roosevelt, the United States Public Health Service was introduced in 1912. During this period assessment of the state of health of newly arrived immigrants in New York was deemed to be of paramount importance. In 1906 Upton Sinclair published a seminal book entitled "The Jungle"[30] which thoroughly described the atrocious lack of hygiene employed continuously in the Chicago Stockyards. This unprecedented expose has been directly credited with the passage of the Pure Food and Drug Act of 1906 which generated new legal requirements for cleanliness of restaurants and food handlers.[31] The new law led to a dramatic reduction in typhoid infections of the intestinal tract-a major cause of serious morbidity with often fatal outcome. Concepts of quarantine and isolation for patients infected with tuberculosis were developed to further reduce spread of communicable disease in the pre-antibiotic era. Although not highly infectious, leprosy could also be controlled by long-term isolation. In 1900 the United States Army sent Major Walter Reed to verify transmission of Yellow Fever by mosquitoes. He showed unequivocally that the vomitus, urine, and feces of yellow fever victims *did not* transmit the disease. He proved definitively that

---

29 Porter, Roy. *The Greatest Benefit to Mankind*. New York, London: Horton and Company, 1997, pp.445-6.

30 Sinclair, Upton. *The Jungle*.1906.

31 *Our Times*. Editor in Chief :Lorraine Glennon, Atlanta: Turner Publishing Inc. p52

the culprit was mosquitoes which spread the virus through a bite of the human skin.[32] Walter Reed and his co-workers proved that drainage of standing water pools along with mosquito netting could dramatically reduce infection born by insect vectors by eliminating breeding grounds.[33] Introduction of these basic hygienic measures by Gorgas allowed construction of the Panama Canal by workers whose ranks had previously been decimated by yellow fever. Today we recognize that insect vectors-mosquitoes in particular-are responsible for greater than one million deaths yearly from malaria worldwide as well as the recent epidemic of Zika virus in the Americas.

The employment of immunization largely seems to have been taken for granted by the mid-twentieth century. Although Jenner had vaccinated against smallpox two centuries previously, it was not until 1949 that widespread immunization in the form of DPT vaccine against diphtheria, whooping cough and tetanus became the standard.[34] In 1955 and 1956 Drs. Sabin and Salk developed immunization against the polio virus essentially eliminating the scourge of infantile paralysis in the USA. Unfortunately this discovery occurred too late for President Franklin Roosevelt who spent most of his adult life in a wheelchair-standing only with great difficulty using braces and crutches. Many children who developed respiratory paralysis spent months in an "iron lung". As a youngster I witnessed children (of friends and neighbors) who had been partially paralyzed by poliovirus infection with varying degrees of recovery. Credit must be due to the epidemiologists, immunologists and public health workers who toiled tirelessly during the early 20th century to control the spread of infectious disease, By the late 1960s a variety of immunizations were required by law for children entering school

---

32 Porter, Roy. *The Greatest Benefit to Mankind*. New York, London: Horton and Company, 1997. pp473-4.

33 Koprowski, Hilary and Michael, B.A. *Microbe Hunters—Then and Now*. Bloomington, Ill: Medi—Ed Press, 1996. pp99-102

34 Porter, Roy. *The Greatest Benefit to Mankind*. New York, London: Horton and Company,1997. p460,485.

or adults enrolling in the military. Finally, children born at that time could be protected from the dangerous risks of pneumonia and encephalitis attributable to measles virus infection.[35] Clearly enormous progress had been made since the time of World War 1 when millions died during a worldwide viral influenza epidemic.

As had been suggested earlier in this volume, progress in surgical treatment had preceded the development of medical therapy available for individual patients. These successes were largely dependent on the advances in antisepsis (hygiene) and anesthesia which have been described in the foregoing pages. The state-of-the-art in the 19th century is clearly reflected in Thomas Eakins' painting entitled "The Gross Clinic" produced around 1876 in Philadelphia. In the portrait surgeons and assistants are dressed in *business suits*. The operating area is in a well-located at the bottom of a large amphitheater where numerous students wearing "street clothes" are seated just above the operating area observing the master surgeon. No gowns, caps or masks are seen nor are there barriers of any type between observers and patient. In contrast, in his painting done about 1889 entitled:" The Agnew Clinic", utilization of surgical gowns is obvious. These are both images of hospitals in Philadelphia which were among the most advanced in the nation. A few years later, during the early 20th century, William Halsted, his assistants and nurses are photographed wearing gowns, caps and gloves in the operating room of the Johns Hopkins Hospital in Baltimore.[36] Halsted had introduced thin rubber gloves into the operating room to protect the skin of Miss Hampton, a nurse who soon became his wife.

Even Halsted, professor and chief of surgery at Johns Hopkins became a victim of one of the greatest of all public health problems which remains unsolved to this day. In contrast to the dramatic

---

35 Koprowski, Hillary. *Microbe Hunters then and now.* Bloomington, Ill Medi-ED Press, 1998, pp70-71

36 Torvald, Jürgen. *The Century of The Surgeon.* New York: Pantheon Books Inc.,1956 (photo preceding p 369)

reduction in communicable disease, addiction to alcohol and opiates continues to present an enormous challenge to physicians and the public. While experimenting with cocaine as a local anesthetic Halsted became forever addicted to this drug.[37] He was placed in formal treatment followed by superb support of William H. Welch, the legendary Hopkins pathologist. Although able to continue in his academic post, the drug habit was never fully conquered.

The Pure Food and Drug Act did require labeling of products and standardization of packaged ingredients. However in the early 20th century most medicines were offered as alcoholic solutions to the patient. In spite of "prohibition "(The Volstead Act), increased consumption of intoxicating liquids became the norm.[38] Although whiskey, gin and similar beverages could be purchased illegally, new dangerous health problems arose as the public discovered cheap alcohol substitutes such as methanol and antifreeze with often fatal results. While the repeal of prohibition in 1935 reduced fatalities following ingestion of toxic alcohol substitutes, opiate addiction flourished-evolving into a major enterprise of organized crime along with prostitution and gambling. Distribution of heroin on the streets of America became a primary income producer for the Mafia. As this addiction and demand for opiates increased, addicts began sharing contaminated needles for injection leading to often fatal infection by HIV and hepatitis virus. Prescription of oral opiate narcotic substitutes only led to increased numbers of addicts, greater health hazards and economic losses persisting into the twenty first century. History of narcotic control is addressed in a later chapter.

Beginning in mid-twentieth-century additional threats to public health developed in relation to widespread recreational ingestion of mind-altering hallucinogens. The disorientation and paranoia produced by compounds such as LSD and PCP led to bizarre

---

[37] Torvald, Jurgen. *The Century of the Surgeon*. New York : Pantheon Books Inc.,1956, p297.

[38] *Our Times*. Editor in Chief :Lorraine Glennon. Atlanta: Turner Publishing Inc.1995. p141, p171, p225

alteration of reality including attempts by individuals to *fly from rooftops*. Although the random shootings at children's schools are often attributed to schizophrenic behavior, hallucinogenic drugs may have produced the culprits in some cases.[39]

In spite of modern advances in basic understanding of infectious mechanisms, global health is severely threatened in the 20th century by deadly viruses such as Ebola which killed thousands in Africa during 2015. Control of transmission by this potentially lethal virus was achieved only by super- intensive quarantine efforts. The world-especially Latin America-is presently engaged in preventing spread of Zika virus which has already produced numerous cases of microcephaly and mental retardation due to infection of pregnant women. Apparently it is transmitted not only by the Aedes Aegypti mosquito bite but also by human sperm. This malady portends disastrous economic and social implications for the coming generation if not rapidly brought under control.

---

39 Katzung, Bertram G. *Basic and Clinical Pharmacology*, Norwalk, Connecticut: Appleton and Lange,1995, pp484-486

Chapter 3

Education

Essential advances in the scientific basis of modern medicine including antisepsis, anesthesia and microbiology had been achieved by the end of the 19th century -particularly in Europe. However dissemination of this knowledge had thus far been restricted largely to a limited number of major medical centers in the United States -including the University of Pennsylvania, Harvard and Johns Hopkins. In this regard it appears that advances in medical treatment lagged well behind the progress in Natural Science e.g. physics and chemistry. Radioactivity and x-ray were identified as early as 1895 and Marconi's Wireless apparatus appeared in 1897 eventually allowing rapid transatlantic communication.

Advances in medicine developed by the previous generation led to a conclusive requirement for improvement in medical education. In 1911 Abraham Flexner produced a report which exposed glaring deficiencies in the medical curriculum. His study described the need for an essential preparation for entrance into medical schools as well as material to be covered following admission. Prior to this time many existing schools functioned as little more than "diploma mills". [40]Pre - medical education beyond high school was not required for entrance until 1898 (Hopkins) and 1900 (Harvard). The majority of non- university affiliated medical courses often granted a degree or license to practice medicine to individuals who had no hospital training whatsoever. These students' education had been limited to a short series of lectures on a variety of topics supplemented by a kind of apprenticeship. The following paragraph describes the basic medical education of John Shaw Billings during 1838-1839 at the Medical college of Ohio. Billings, who served as a battlefield surgeon during the Civil War later became an assistant Surgeon General. His medical education consisted of two full courses of lectures each identical in content lasting from four to five months during the winters of two successive years. The lecture schedule continued six days per week for eight hours daily. The courses *were not* graded. Hospital instruction was given for 2 hours weekly. Following these lectures he served one year as a resident physician in a hospital in Cincinnati for indigent and mentally disadvantaged individuals.[41] The most important result of Flexner's report was the reduction in total number of medical schools from 133 in 1890 to 85 in 1920. In many cases the physicians who now staffed the hospitals were employed as professors by the affiliated university.[42]

In addition to reorganization of the professional staff and marked lengthening of the standard medical curriculum was the introduction of scientific journals such as JAMÀ and "Surgery Gynecology and Obstetrics" introduced by John F. Martin which first appeared in July 1905.[43] This publication which has endured throughout the 20th

---

40 Flexner, Abraham *Medical Education in the United States and Canada*. Boston: Marymount Press, 1910.

41 Chapman, Carleton B. *Order out of Chaos*. New York:Carleton Chapman Science History Publications/USA. pp.37-39.

42 Flexner, Abraham. *Medical Education in the United States and Canada Boston: Marymount Press.1910.*

43 American College of Surgeons: *Remembering Milestones and achievements in Surgery*. Tampa, Florida : Fairmount Media 2012. p66.

century was edited by surgical luminaries of the period including Nicholas Senn, John B Murphy, Franklin Martin and Allen B. Kanavel of Chicago. Surgical contributors were drawn from the entire nation.

In an effort to improve teaching of clinical medicine and patient care Billings and Gilman devised a plan for the new Johns Hopkins Hospital and medical school which opened in 1887. This institution employed a full-time staff composed of professors of medicine, surgery, obstetrics etc. from the medical school. The Hopkins plan, unusual for the time, encouraged teaching and research in academic medicine in contrast to full-time fee for service patient care. An alternative at certain institutions was to place the faculty on a part time salary allowing private practice to supplement their income from teaching.[44]

Within a year of his attachment to Halsted's surgical staff, Harvey Cushing assumed responsibility in addition to patient care, surgery etc. for the Hunterian laboratory --instructing third-year medical students in the anatomy and techniques of surgery. This course remained one of Cushing's top priorities during the next 12 years prior to his acceptance of the Mosley professorship of surgery (in 1911) at the Harvard Medical School.[45] Organization and standardization of medical instruction helped to provide a certain level of assurance to the public that they were no longer to be subjected to quackery or fraud by poorly trained individuals. By 1918 it was clearly recognized that medical practice additionally required enhancement and regulation of hospital standards. A survey of hospitals contaning at least 104 beds by the American College of Surgeons(founded 1913) showed that only 12% of 692 institutions reviewed met a set

---

44 Chapman, Carleton B. *Order out of Chaos*. New York: Carleton B. Chapman Science History Publications/USA.

45 Fulton, John Farquhar. *Harvey Cushing, a Biography*. Springfield: Charles C Thomas.1945.

of "minimum standards of care".[46] A program requiring 5 years of hospital training for surgical specialist certification was constructed by the College.

Careful review of medical and surgical admissions and discharges by hospital staff would provide an important stimulus to enhanced graduate medical education and improved patient outcome. By the 1950's standardized testing following the second and fourth years of medical schools school had been developed by the National Board of Medical Examiners. In Illinois a third part of the examination which included an oral session was required after one year of hospital internship in order to obtain a license to practice medicine. Subsequently, continuing medical education through courses and meetings became the norm for maintaining certification for licensure.

---

46 American College of Surgeons: *Remembering Milestones and achievements in Surgery*. Tampa, Florida : Fairmount Media, 2012.

Chapter 4

Physiology

While great strides in defining the details of post-mortem tissues and microbial agents had been made by the nineteenth and early twentieth century by pathologists such as Virchow, Koch and Welch, major improvements in therapy were made possible by contributions of the physiologists who studied the living body. Critical contributions in regard to the dynamic functions of several tissues and organs were made by the great French physiologist Claude Bernard during the 18 th century. In particular he studied blood oxygenation, and neurologic control of small blood vessels and the action of curare at the nerve- muscle junction. Of paramount importance was his discovery of pancreatic digestive enzymes and the critical conversion of glucose to glycogen by the liver.[47]

Although the basic concepts of circulation and blood volume were seen to be essential for life, very little was known in regard to hormonal control (endocrinology) of body functions. Even less was understood in regard to the role of the nervous system although it was now clear that epileptic seizures were secondary to dysfunction of the cerebral cortex. When one considers that the human body

---

47 Porter, Roy. *The Greatest Benefit to Mankind*. New York, London: Horton and Company, 1997, p19.

is effectively under the control of the nervous system, then an understanding of neurophysiology appears of paramount importance in the maintenance of human health. During his year of European study in 1901, while awaiting appointment to Halsted's surgical staff, Harvey Cushing made an astounding discovery. He found that blood pressure rose and pulse rate slowed in response to increased intracranial pressure. Working in Berne(Kronecker's laboratory) Cushing observed this phenomenon by direct visualization of a dog's brain through an opening in the skull. It was apparent that defense of brain perfusion (blood flow) and function is maintained by alteration of general body hemodynamics through the nervous system.[48]

Technical and theoretical advances in general and organic chemistry laid the foundation for biochemical determinations essential to the practice of modern medicine. In the 1880s Ringer had been evaluating the application of physiologic saline to living tissue. In Berne, Switzerland (Kocher's clinic), Cushing determined that neuro muscular function could not be sustained by a solution composed only of sodium chloride. He found that physiologic solutions required limited amounts of potassium and calcium ions for the continuation of neural activity.[49]

In 1907 Donald Van Slyke, an experienced chemist, joined the Rockefeller Institute for medical research. By the end of World War 1 he had developed a method for precisely measuring blood gases including oxygen and carbon dioxide in human blood. Quantitative assessment of these substances for the first time allowed the physician to recognize the condition of metabolic acidosis, a critical assessment in a variety of diseases -especially in diabetes. It was not until 1931 that Peters and van Slyke collaborated on the publication of a classic volume entitled "Quantitative Clinical Chemistry"[50] which set

---

48 Fulton, John Farquhar. *Harvey Cushing, a Biography*. Springfield: Charles C. Thomas,1946.

49 Fulton, John Farquhar. *Harvey Cushing, a Biography* Springfield: Charles C. Thomas,1946

50 Peters, John P. and Van Slyke Donald. *Quantitative Clinical Chemistry,1932*.

important standards for hospital laboratories regarding renal function and blood chemical homeostasis.

According to Fulton, Harvey Cushing had developed an extensive *interest in physiology during his early years as Halsted's assistant at* Hopkins. In addition to General Surgery and experimental work in physiology performed at the Hunterian laboratory, he had been assigned the responsibility for neurological cases presenting to the Hopkins surgical department.[51]

Certainly a portion of the progress in neurophysiology at this time was the byproduct of neurosurgical intervention. Around 1901 Charles Fraser in Philadelphia began to surgically treat trigeminal neuralgia.[52] Cushing operated on a series of patients of which a number required excision or destruction of the Gasserian ganglion at the skull base to relieve trigeminal neuralgia. This surgical approach inevitably led to more detailed appreciation of the sensory innervation of the face and forehead as well as the dental structures. Gradual experience with cranial surgery during this period led W.W. Keen of Philadelphia (who had successfully removed a brain tumor during the 1880's) to ask Cushing to write a chapter on neurological surgery for his classic treatise on surgery. It was at this time that physiology of the endocrine glands controlled by the pituitary body began to be understood.

Apparently Frolich (1901) had studied the case of a young woman whose clinical picture was exemplified by adiposity, lethargy and underdeveloped genital organs of which Cushing became aware. The diagnosis in this case proved to be a pituitary gland tumor.[53] Cushing subsequently encountered a similar case at Hopkins which he operated upon unsuccessfully. He described the details of this

---

51 Fulton, John Farquhar. *Harvey Cushing A Biography*. Springfield: Charles C. Thomas, 1945, p216-220.

52 Fulton, John Farquhar. *Harvey Cushing, A Biography*. Springfield: Charles C. Thomas, 1945, pp264-5.

53 Fulton, John Farquhar. *Harvey Cushing, A Biography*. Springfield: Charles C. Thomas, 1945, pp. 271-2.

patient's case in 1901 and subsequently focused a great deal of effort on understanding the role of the hypophysis (pituitary body) in health and disease. Following the successful excision of a large hypophyseal tumor in an acromegalic individual, Cushing published several papers based on a series of about 50 pituitary tumors which were referred to him between 1910 and 1912.[54] Additionally much effort was devoted to experimental hypophysectomy in dogs through work in the Hunterian laboratory at Hopkins. Cushing recognized the critical relationship between the pituitary and endocrine glands including the adrenals, gonads and thyroid.[55] A Nobel Prize in physiology and Medicine (1950) was awarded to Kendall for his elucidation of the chemical structure of the adrenal hormone, cortisone, which proved dramatically effective in the treatment of rheumatoid arthritis. Additional research demonstrated the critical importance of aldosterone (also an adrenal product) in the maintenance of salt and water balance in the body. Through his experimental work on dogs Cushing recognized the important but separate secretions of hormones by the posterior portion of the pituitary body -in particular the antidiuretic hormone.

Little attention to the fundamental importance of blood volume seems to have been paid in review of the development of surgery. However Alfred Blaylock of Johns Hopkins provided a beginning understanding of "shock" in 1927. By 1934 Blaylock was able to describe "shock" as the result of a decrease in the ratio of blood volume to the capacity of the vascular bed. This situation clearly underlies the fall in blood pressure seen in wounding/hemorrhage, sepsis, and extensive burns. In 1949 it was shown that a dramatic

---

54 Fulton, John Farquhar. *Harvey Cushing, A Biography*. Springfield: Charles C. Thomas, 1945, p p299-304.

55 Porter, Roy) *The Greatest Benefit to Mankind*. New York, London: Horton and Company,1997. p566

increase in survival occurred in patients in shock when large volumes of Lactated Ringer's solution were added to the resuscitating fluid. [56]

Although Landsteiner had described blood types A B and C (later called type AB) as early as 1900, direct transfusions from patient to patient developed by Carrel in 1908, were still in use at the time of World War I. Hektoen introduced cross matching to preclude transfusion reaction in 1907. Specifically there were no adequate methods of storage until the introduction of citrate by Levisohn around 1914.[57] Accurate measurement of blood volume was not clinically utilized until well after World War II. Estimation of blood loss is especially difficult in cases of battlefield wounding. Recognition of this fundamental dilemma led to empirical administration of plasma (not requiring refrigeration) to the recently wounded prior to evacuation from the battlefield during WWII.

An additional area of human physiology of considerable importance had developed since the early 19th century through the observations of William Beaumont. As a physician he had cared for Alexis St. Martin who suffered a permanent gastric fistula following an abdominal gunshot wound. Beaumont was able to directly observe gastric digestion in the partially exposed stomach (over a period of years) through his continued treatment of this individual in the last part of the 19th century.[58]. Much of what was known in regard to gastrointestinal physiology at that time was gleaned through abdominal surgery. In a sense the normal physiology was discovered and understood as pathological conditions were explored. More detailed presentation of this aspect will be described in conjunction with our discussion of progress in clinical surgery. The relationship between the reflex activity of the stomach and the central nervous

---

56 Millham, Frederick Heaton. "A Brief History of Shock". *Surgery*, vol148, no.5, 2010, pp1026-1037.

57 Giangrande, Paul. L.F. "The History of Blood Transfusions". *British Journal of Haematology*, 2000, vol.110, p758-767.

58 Porter, Roy. *The Greatest Benefit to Mankind*. New York, London: Horton and Company,1997.

system was demonstrated by Ivan Pavlov who conditioned dogs to salivate at the sound of a bell. His experimental work furthered understanding of the intimate relationship between the brain and peripheral nervous system.[59]

Understanding the essential mechanism of kidney function is credited to E.K. Marshal Jr of Johns Hopkins. By chance this outstanding physiologist/ pharmacologist happened to be a next-door neighbor of my grandparents in Baltimore. Dr. Marshall unequivocally demonstrated that the human kidney filters, reabsorbs and secretes fluid and electrolytes to maintain homeostasis in the blood. He subsequently held the chair of physiology and later Pharmacology at Johns Hopkins where his fundamental research was carried out. During the decade preceding WWll he also successfully investigated. the action of Sulfonamides in the treatment of infection.

---

59 Porter, Roy. *The Greatest Benefit to Mankind*. New York, London: Horton and Company.1997, pp544-545.

CHAPTER 5

Part 1: Dr. Cushing's War

It is often stated that "chance favors the prepared mind". Harvey Cushing had the advantage of a strong, well educated, financially secure family which allowed him to study at Yale College and the Harvard Medical School from which he graduated in 1896. Cushing's intellectual curiosity and indefatigability enabled him to make discoveries of profound significance as a very young man. Two of these innovations have already been described: first, the introduction of the ether chart for anesthesia[60] and subsequently the "Cushing reflex" in which blood pressure rises concomitantly with increasing intracranial pressure.[61] During the next decade and a half prior to the onset of World War 1 he operated upon a series of brain tumors with increasing success and decreasing mortality and morbidity. During this period Cushing had the advantage of clear understanding of aseptic technique, general anesthesia and operating in a field which would not be contaminated by the procedure. Abdominal surgeons entering the gastrointestinal tract were not afforded that luxury.

---

60 Fulton, John Farquhar. *Harvey Cushing, a Biography*. Springfield: Charles C. Thomas,1945, pp93-6.

61 Fulton, John Farquhar. *Harvey Cushing, a Biography*. Springfield: Charles C. Thomas,1945, p184.

Utilizing the meticulous surgical technique he had learned from Halsted at the Hopkins, Cushing begin to remove brain tumors with increasing success. By 1914 - 15 he had done a hundred and fifty craniotomies with a mortality of 7% while the mortality recently reported from the National Hospital at Queen Square indicated a mortality near 50%.

Following twelve years at Johns Hopkins, Harvey Cushing was appointed surgeon –in chief at the Peter Bent Brigham in Boston. During the fifth year as Mosley professor of surgery at Harvard, Cushing determined to support the Allies in Europe by organizing a hospital unit to serve in France. Having obtained the support of the Brigham hospital's directors he sailed from Boston with a surgical team and support staff on March 18th, 1915. Following a stormy journey to Gibraltar they traveled via Madrid to Bordeaux, where Cushing observed that "the majority of the men were admitted to hospital at Neuilly with bronchitis and influenza-like colds".[62] During the early days things were badly disorganized and the conditions were shocking. The wounded were all rushed out as rapidly as possible and the more seriously ill we're put off wherever and whenever the train stopped. They were picked up in any way chance might favor --luckily if by an ambulance but more often by a cattle or provision train returning from the Front. One of these trains had dumped about 500 badly wounded men and left them lying between tracks in the rain with no cover whatsoever.[63] One can only conclude that very little progress in evacuation had been achieved since the Crimean and American Civil War. Cushing further recorded "we were informed that the medical situation was improving since there were only 500 cases of typhoid fever in the 4000 beds at Amiens". Typhoid apparently carried at least a 13% mortality. An investigation of the trenches revealed these ditches extended all the way from

---

62 Cushing, H.C. *From a Surgeons Journal 1915-1918*. Boston: Little Brown and Company.1936.

63 Fulton, John Farquhar. *Harvey Cushing, a Biography*. Springfield: Charles C.. Thomas, p395.

Flanders to Switzerland. "....strange warfare fit only for moles, weasel and rats......" One may be reminded of Hemingway's experiences as an ambulance driver as Cushing described the "Service de Santé".

The following quotation by Fulton from Cushing's WW1 diary gives a clear picture of the conditions which were encountered by the Brigham's surgeons. He described. "The amazing patience of the seriously wounded-some of them hanging on for months... the dreadful deformities; the tedious healing of the infected wounds with discharging sinuses, tubes, irrigations, and repeated dressings so much so that grating and painful fractures are simply abandoned to wait for wounds to heal which they don't seem to do. ...the risks under apparently favorable circumstances of attempting clean operations most of which seem to have broken down-A varicocele and appendix and worst of all a thoracotomy for a bullet in the pericardium which apparently was doing no harm".

Prior to his return home in May 1916, Cushing experienced the results of a "gas attack" at Ypres-in this instance chlorine. The number and severity of casualties was appalling. After returning to Boston, he organized an American Army unit (base hospital # 5) which sailed for Europe in April 1917 following America's entry into the war. Cushing again describes the hygiene and public health aspects of war including infestation with lice (transmitting typhus) and scabies as well as epidemics of measles and mumps. Additionally on Sept 4, 1917 his hospital was bombed. Undeterred, Dr. Cushing reported a series of 119 brain wounds-the detailed records of which were utilized to advantage at the outset of WW II. Finally in August 1918, having been promoted to the rank of Lt. Colonel, he personally sustained an acute neurological disorder which impaired his mobility and was most likely Guillen-Barre syndrome.[64] Of corollary interest is that of the 326,000 casualties only half were related to wounding in battle. Surprisingly, these figures had changed little since the American Civil War!

---

64 Fulton, John Farquhar. *Harvey Cushing, a Biography*. Springfield: Charles C. Thomas,1945, p435.

Following the war period, during which millions died of the complications of influenza, Milton Winternitz (trained by Welch at Hopkins) undertook a massive study of pulmonary pathology in these cases which showed edema and bronchiolar obstruction leading to a fatal outcome. Description of the effects of Phosgene gas released by the Germans at Ypres and other sites showed the lungs filling with secreted fluid within a few hours-virtually a death by drowning!

Keegan's treatise describes the wartime experiences of Edwin Vaughn, an officer of the first Warwickshire regiment : "up the road we staggered, shells bursting around us ; a man stopped dead in front of me and exasperated I cursed him and butted him with my knee. Very gently he said 'I'm blind sir 'and turned to show me his eyes and nose torn away by a piece of shell. A tank had turned slowly behind and opened fire. A moment later I looked and nothing remained of it but a crumpled heap of iron-it had been hit by a large shell,". "From other shell holes from the darkness on all sides came the groans and wails of wounded men, long shopping moans of agony and despairing shrieks. It was too horribly obvious that dozens of men with serious wounds must have crawled for safety into new shell holes and now the water was rising about them and powerless to move they were slowly drowning".[65]

---

65 Keegan, John *The First World War.* New York: Alfred A. Knopf,1999.

Chapter 5

Part 2: Principles of Wound care and Outcome

W.W. Keen M.D., an outstanding American surgeon who had first served in the Civil War described the advanced techniques of wound management derived from the experience of surgeons during WWI. His book "Treatment of War Wounds" published in 1917 describes clearly the progress in treatment gleaned by using knowledge of bacteriology in the control of infection. A description of a wound caused by shell fragments notes the critical importance of thorough debridement to remove pieces of newspaper, clothing, and gravel. He further points out that "... the soil which contaminates these wounds contains in addition to the usual pyogenic bacteria-- soil impregnated with the virulent fecal bacteria, derived from unsanitary conditions of trench life". Carrel, a French surgeon, had observed that when a wound was examined bacteriologically as early as six hours after infection --bacteria were few in number and localized around the muscle. Twenty-four hours later bacteria were found everywhere. Considerable attention is devoted to Dakin's solution:(sodium hypochlorite) which is bactericidal. Detailed instructions are given for production of the antiseptic in the field hospital by Dakin and Carrel. Further description is given of an ingenious system of tubing which is introduced into the wound for constant irrigation designed to eradicate bacteria.[66] Keen notes that "the two most important witnesses are unquestionably Professor William H. Welch and Professor Depage. The testimony of Professor William H. Welch of Johns Hopkins is most valuable because of his eminence as a pathologist and as a broad-minded philosophic observer". Following a visit to the (WWI) medical facilities at Compiegne during which he studied the method and the smears "day by day", Welch concluded "there can be no question that Carrel deserves the credit…of recalling the attention of surgeons to the possibility of the sterilization of infected wounds by chemical means….that the Carrel-Dakin procedure actually accomplishes such sterilization sufficiently for surgical purposes is *conclusively demonstrated*".[67] The efficacy of such treatment was shown by a group of 80 compound fractures which exhibited no pus on the dressings. It is worth noting that while tetanus was in general a rarity, the not uncommon case during the American Civil War carried a mortality of 89%. Marked reduction in mortality during WWI is attributed to the availability of tetanus antiserum and the previously described management of wounds.

Control of typhoid fever reflects one of the most important advances from a medical standpoint. The Financial secretary for the British War Ministry stated that there were only 4571 cases in the whole army thorough November 1917 compared with 1 case for every 5 soldiers during the Spanish-American war of 1898. This figure is attributed to careful supervision of the water supply. Finally it is noted that the operative mortality from abdominal wounds lay at 53%, considered a significant improvement on the non-operative treatment during the Boer War where mortality was near 100%.

---

66   Keen, W.W. *The Treatment of War Wounds*. Philadelphia and London: WB. Saunders company,1918, p88-103

67   Keen, W.W. *The Treatment of War Wounds*. Philadelphia and London:W.B. Saunders company,1918, p79-81

Chapter 6

The End of the beginning

William Halsted has frequently been considered historically to have been the father of American surgery. Born in 1852 he graduated from Yale College in 1874. After obtaining his M.D. from Columbia Medical School in New York City, he interned at the Bellevue Hospital. First established in 1736, a similar institution- Philadelphia General Hospital (originally Friends almshouse) had emerged to provide care for indigent war veterans and immigrants. From New York Halsted travelled to Vienna where Theodor Billroth had developed advanced general surgical techniques. After operating successfully at various New York City hospitals, Halsted was offered the position of chief of surgery at Johns Hopkins by Welch in 1890. He then became professor of surgery, part of the first full-time medical faculty at Hopkins.[68]

By the turn of the century critical advances in general surgery had been achieved in Europe most notably by Billroth and Mikulicz in Vienna, Kocher in Berne and von Bergman in Germany. In the late 1880s Billroth had pioneered an operation (subtotal gastrectomy) which allowed excision of a portion of the stomach harboring

---

68 Porter, Roy. *The Greatest Benefit to Mankind*. New York, London: Horton and Company, 1997. p604.

cancer [69] and reconnecting the remaining gastrointestinal tract. Partial gastric excision then also became available for treatment of peptic ulcer and other non-malignant conditions. During this period, aided by general anesthesia and antisepsis, Halsted was able to perform radical mastectomy designed to cure previously fatal cases of breast cancer. He also developed an effective repair of inguinal hernia.[70] The most difficult and challenging area of general surgery lay in dealing with peritonitis, a diffuse spread of infection into the general abdominal cavity which inevitably led to death. By far the most common cause of acute peritonitis was inflammation and subsequent rupture of the vermiform appendix attached to the cecum. During the last decade of the nineteenth century Reginald Fitz, a pathologist, described the condition now called appendicitis and strongly advocated its surgical removal prior to rupture.[71] It became apparent to several pioneer surgeons including Mc Burney in New York and John B. Murphy in Chicago that early diagnosis and excision of the inflamed appendix would save many lives. Appendectomy became the most common operation and ultimately important advance in general surgery at the onset of the 20th century. Shortly thereafter safe excision of the inflamed gallbladder (cholecystectomy) was achieved.[72] A review of several sources suggested that at the time of Harvey Cushing's transfer to the Brigham hospital in Boston from Johns Hopkins (around 1911 / 1912), the majority of basic advances in general surgery occurring prior to the 1930's had been achieved. Although the coronation of Edward the seventh of England was of necessity temporarily

---

69 Torvald, Jurgen. *The Century of the Surgeon*. New York: Pantheon Books, 1956, pp342-349.

70 Halsted, W.H. "The Radical Cure of Inguinal Hernia in the Male". *Bull. Johns Hopkins hospital*, vol.4, no.29, Mar, 1893, pp.17-24.

71 Porter, Roy. *The Greatest Benefit to Mankind*. New York, London: Horton and Company, 1997, pp.361-363.

72

postponed in 1902, his life was saved by an appendectomy performed in London by Sir Frederick Treves.[73]

In 2012 the American College of surgeons published an remarkable summary of its first 100 years. The sobering data which follows illustrates the limitations of surgical success which persisted near the advent of WWII. Dr. David Richardson cites a report of 755 cases of appendectomy in New York in 1929 having a 6.3% operative mortality. In a group of patients 51 years or older 25% died. An incredible mortality of 42% was documented for appendectomy in those over 60! A report of 500 cholecystectomies (gallbladder removal) from Memphis, Tennessee yielded a 4% death rate while more than one in ten failed to survive gastric resection in a series reported in 1939.[74] Such statistics would have been appalling by the late 1950's when I was enrolled at Yale.

A 1950 review of patients requiring <u>emergency</u> surgery (surgery unrelated to trauma) described 17% mortality. Following commonly performed operations for conditions such as bowel obstruction, appendicitis, cholecystitis and amputation of an extremity for gangrene in patients over 60 years of age nearly 40% died. On a far more positive note, Dr. Carl Moyer of the Barnes Hospital in St. Louis showed that overall mortality for appendectomy had declined to 0.7% by 1950. The dramatic improvement was attributed to 1) safer anesthesia 2) understanding of fluid and electrolyte balance 3) antibiotics and 4) intensive care units.

Following several anecdotal excisions of brain tumors by Durante (1884) Rickman Godlee (1886) and W.W. Keen in Philadelphia, (1887) [75] the pioneering success of brain surgery is attributable to Harvey Cushing. Prior to his move to Boston as Mosley professor at

---

[73] Torvald, Jurgen. *The Century of the Surgeon*. New York: Pantheon Books, 1953, p53.

[74] American College of Surgeons: *Remembering Milestones and achievements in Surgery*. Tampa, Florida: Fairmount Media Group, 2012, pp45-46.

[75] Fulton, John Farquhar. *Harvey Cushing, A. Biography*. Springfield:CharlesC. Thomas,1946.

the newly-opened Brigham hospital he had operated on an extensive series of pituitary and, cerebral tumors, as well as growths in the posterior cranial fossa.[76] His success was all the more remarkable since it was achieved in the absence of antibiotics, banked blood for transfusion, and general endotracheal anesthesia. Meanwhile a second neurosurgical genius had arisen from the Johns Hopkins medical Class of 1911. Walter Dandy from Missouri spent the next seven years as assistant resident and resident to William Halstead finally completing his training in 1918. His greatest contribution to neurophysiology and surgery was achieved in 1913 when he (with Blackfan) described the circulation of cerebrospinal fluid from the ventricles of the brain (where it was formed) into the spinal canal and subsequently returned to the brain surface for reabsorption.[77] Near the end of WWI Dandy introduced the radiographic technique which long-term Cushing assistant Gilbert Horrax believed had increased the diagnosis and localization of brain tumors by at least 30%. Dandy had become familiar with the value of gas/air abdominal x-rays by this time. He astutely realized that similar contrast studies could be achieved following the introduction of air into the ventricles of the brain. Dandy now developed the procedure of ventriculography which could show displacement of brain tissue by a tumor or mass on an x-ray plate. Finally in 1922 Dandy published a series of tumors (acoustic neuromas) which he had totally excised from the cerebellopontine angle preventing recurrence.[78] Walter Dandy remained the singular neurosurgeon at Johns Hopkins (although he trained many younger men), until his death in 1946.

---

[76] Fulton, John Farquhar *Harvey Cushing, a Biography*, Springfield: Charles C. Thomas, p299,301,321

[77] American College of Surgeons: *Remembering Milestones and achievements in Surgery*. Tampa, Florida : Fairmount Media Group, 2012

[78] Fulton, John Farquhar. *Harvey Cushing, a Biography*. Springfield: Charles C. Thomas,1946, p490.

Chapter 7

Radiology: A great leap forward in medical diagnosis

The discovery of x-Rays by Wilhelm Roentgen during the last decade of the 19th century provided the physician with an opportunity to view parts of the interior of the human body from without. One could now confirm suspected bony fractures, infection, osteomyelitis, pneumonia, and tumors as well as more benign joint pathology designated "arthritis". While bone fractures had been known for centuries and other bone lesions had been confirmed more recently by pathologists, it was now possible to achieve a definitive diagnosis in the living patient. The presence of air and gas contrast in radiographs was recognized early in the twentieth century enabling the radiologist to identify lesions of varying density in the lung. One could now differentiate between an inflammatory process (such as tuberculosis or pneumonia.[79]) and lesions of lung cancer, emphysema, or pulmonary edema. Having seen early utilization of X-ray while a student at Harvard, Cushing had introduced its application to medicine at Johns Hopkins by the turn of the century.

---

79 Porter, Roy. *The Greatest Benefit to Mankind.* New York, London: Horton and Company, 1997.

At the present time (2018) there are more than 100,000 new cases of colon cancer discovered each year. Twenty-five percent of these malignancies prove fatal. Examination of the gastrointestinal tract was advanced by introduction of opaque contrast material. A solution of bismuth sub nitrate was employed in 1904 by Schule while Haenich reported a bismuth enema accompanied by fluoroscopy in 1911. Utilizing these methods colonic tumors were identified in 1923 by Carman and Fineman. Improved detail in radiography of colonic lesions was achieved utilizing colloidal barium sulfate in the 1940s. Manual compression of the abdomen during the examination was introduced to delineate polyps obscured by layers of Barium. Micro pulverized suspensions of Barium were utilized beginning in the 1950's. Demonstration of non-opaque gallstones (Cholecystogram) by Evarts Graham and Warren Cole appeared in 1924. During recent years evaluation of the colon by CT (computerized tomography) and direct fibreoptic colonoscopy has largely replaced the barium enema. Clearly radiologic evaluation of the colon represents a major advance in the evolution of human healthcare.[80]

Although Harvey Cushing had developed superior surgical techniques for operations on the brain and spine by the end of WWI, [81]precise localization of intracranial lesions remained unsatisfactory until the radiologic techniques of ventriculography and pneumoencephalography were introduced by Walter Dandy around 1919.[82] By introduction of air into the fluid spaces of the brain, displacement of the ventricular system by space occupying lesions could be observed radiographically allowing accurate placement of craniotomy. Further advances in neuroradiology arrived with the introduction of angiography in 1927 although this procedure's

---

80 Levine, Mark S., M.D. and Yee, Judy. "History of Evolution and Current Status of tests for colorectal cancer screening". *Radiology*: vol. 273, number2 (suppl), Nov. 2014.

81 Fulton, John Farquhar. *Harvey Cushing, a Biography*. Springfield: Charles C. Thomas. p305

82 *American College of Surgeons: Remembering Milestones and achievements in Surgery*. Tampa, Florida : Fairmount Media Group, 2012, p133

widespread use was delayed for another decade until a safer contrast material was developed. By injecting a radiopaque substance into an artery in the neck one could visualize cerebral vasculature. Demonstration of brain blood vessels provided identification and localization of tumors, aneurysms, arteriovenous malformations, and compressive blood clots (hematomas).[83] These methods remained the basic radiologic approach until the 1970s when computerized tomography(CT scanning) was introduced. By injecting contrast material(Pantopaque} into the spinal canal one could accurately localize herniated discs and spinal tumors by X-ray prior to surgery[84] which largely eliminated the extensive exploratory laminectomies (spine operations} employed in the first quarter of the 20th century. Clearly angiography became a sine qua non for the introduction and development of carotid endarterectomy to be addressed in a later chapter.

---

[83] *American College of Surgeons: Remembering Milestones and achievements in Surgery.* Tampa, Florida : Fairmount Media Group,2012, p123.

[84] Siqueira, Edir B., Bucy, Paul C. and Cannon, Abram H. "Positive Contrast Ventriculography, Cisternography and Myelography." *American J. Radiology*, vol.104, Sept, 1968, p1-7.

Chapter 8

Immunology: the viral scourge

Long before the essential complex scientific basis for immunity had been explored in the laboratory, Jenner proved that protective immunity against smallpox could be obtained in human beings by inoculation with cowpox. Beginning in the 16th century European explorers had introduced smallpox to the Americas with devastating results. By the eighteenth century it had become endemic in the major cities of Europe. The disease continued to spread throughout the world- killing over 300 million people. Smallpox is a distinctly human disease without a known animal reservoir--highly infectious from person to person. It apparently originated in China and India and was introduced into Europe by the Crusades. Although partly successful attempts at immunization had been achieved in the eleventh and twelfth centuries in the Far East, the modern approach to vaccination was not developed by Jenner until the 1790s.[85] Originally vaccination was obtained by direct arm to arm passage between human subjects. Finally a vaccine was developed in cows in the mid-19th century.

---

85 [85] Porter, Roy. *The Greatest Benefit to Mankind*. New York, London: Horton and Company, 1997.

By May, 1980 it was possible to affirm that the disease had been eradicated throughout the World.[86]

While successful immunization against smallpox and rabies had been achieved by the end of the nineteenth century research was then undertaken to develop a vaccine which would be effective against the bacteria pneumococcus. In 1930 Tillet and then Finland demonstrated that purified polysaccharide capsule of the bacteria offered an opportunity to create some protection. A hexavalent vaccine against multiple pneumococcal strains was introduced in 1946.[87] Unfortunately the effort was largely abandoned due to the introduction of antibiotics at that time. Work continued to develop a pneumococcal vaccine for infants in the late 20th century.

The remainder of this chapter will consider successful development of immunization against the virus of yellow fever, measles, hepatitis and influenza. All of the above have produced extensive morbidity and mortality in World populations and are not susceptible to antibiotic therapy. Reference has previously been made the outstanding efforts of Walter Reed and Gorgas to control yellow fever before the first World War. The disease was apparently initially recognized in the Yucatan of Mexico during the 17th century. In 1828 28% of the inhabitants of New Orleans died of this malady. Tragically one of Reed's young co-workers became infected and died in 1900 after allowing himself to be bitten. Although yellow fever could be controlled in urban areas, the jungle reservoir of the virus could not be eradicated due to monkey infection. Max Theiler and co-workers developed 17D. Vaccine in 1932. Thieler and co-workers were finally awarded a Nobel Prize for their outstanding work in 1951.[88]

---

86 Koprowski, Hillary. *Microbe Hunters Then and Now.* Bloomington, Ill: Medi-Ed Press1996.

87 Koprowski, Hillary. *Microbe Hunters then and now.* Bloomington, Ill Medi-Ed Press1996.

88 Koprowski, Hillary. *Microbe Hunters then and now.* Bloomington, Ill : Medi-Ed Press,1996, pp95-110.

Reference was made to the *polio* virus (in chapter 2) in conjunction with Franklin Roosevelt. The historical description of individuals with withered limbs suggested evidence of the disease in ancient times. Little interest appeared in the medical community until the nineteenth century when a series of cases usually called "infantile paralysis "appeared on St. Helena Island best known as. Napoleon Bonaparte's final place of exile. By 1909 researchers had achieved a major breakthrough when the polio virus was found transmissible to monkeys, allowing experimental work required for a vaccine to proceed. Sadly vaccination with formalin inactivated vaccine yielded several cases of paralytic polio in New York in 1935. Another vaccination attempt using a suspension of infected monkey spinal cord resulted in 12 cases of paralytic polio with six deaths. By 1949 John Enders had cultivated poliovirus in human tissue.[89] Successful immunization was finally achieved in the 1950s. Salk produced a killed vaccine in 1953 which required multiple injections. Koprowski and others' efforts eventually led to the oral vaccination of 244,000 people in the Belgian Congo in 1958 with 68% protection in some groups. Finally statistics obtained for 1992 to 1994 in the United States and Canada yielded 0 cases of polio.[90]

Measles is known to be one of the most contagious diseases on the planet. It has been estimated that this agent infects 16 million individuals yearly with a mortality of 10%. During the 19th century it became clear that measles rapidly spread through large groups such as encampments of soldiers during the American Civil War.[91] Susceptibility is significantly increased by malnutrition and overcrowding. During the first half of the 20th century measles

---

89 Porter, Roy. *The Greatest Benefit to Mankind.* New York, London: Horton and Company,1997 p86.

90 Koprowski, Hillary. *Microbe Hunters Then and Now.* Bloomington, Ill : Medi-Ed Press,1996, pp141-149.

91 Denney Robert. *Civil War Medicine: Care and Comfort of the Wounded.* New York: Sterling Publishing Co.1994, p41,54,60, 61.

was considered one of the most common and expected diseases of childhood in well developed nations. Although those infected were often temporarily quite ill with rash and fever, recovery was normally expected. By the 1960s various complications of measles including pneumonia, otitis media and gastroenteritis were well-known. Additionally the neurologists were confronted by children with post- infectious encephalitis. Following the development of a safe vaccine which was licensed in 1963 the annual number of reported cases in the United States fell from more than 2 million to less than 400 in1995. By this time Global vaccination efforts had reduced childhood deaths around the world from Two and a half million to 750,000.[92]

During the decade of the 1950's relatively little information regarding viral illness was disseminated to medical students. Courses in Microbiology dealt primarily with bacterial, fungal, and protozoan causes of human disease. Common childhood exanthema such as measles, chicken pox and rubella were dismissed as standard features of "growing up". Immunization for polio virus had first been introduced in the mid-fifties and long-term results were yet undetermined. From the standpoint of medical history little attention seemed to be given to the fact that 20-30 million people had died worldwide following infection during the *influenza* pandemic of 1918-1919. In fact this number far exceeded deaths from bubonic or pneumonic plague during the 14th century. An outbreak of the "Asian flu" in 1957 and again in 1968 stimulated intensified research to develop effective vaccines. At this time neither the Ebola or HIV virus had been identified as human pathogens. At one time it was believed that the severe mortality from influenza was solely the result of secondary bacterial infection. Present day evidence indicates that a major culprit is an over-reactive immune response (virus-triggered) which attacks the host (patient's) cells causing widespread injury to normal tissues and organs.

---

92 Koprowski, Hillary. *Microbe Hunters Then and Now*. Bloomington, Ill : Medi-ED Press,1996, pp69-74.

"Through most of the 19th century respiratory illness was generally classified as tubercular or non-tubercular pneumonia". McCullers reported that the H1N1 1918 pandemic influenza strain killed more than 40 million people worldwide and that 95 % of fatal cases were complicated by secondary bacterial infection. In contrast the H3N2 pandemic killed only around one million people. The question was raised as to whether one was dealing with one identical disease process.[93] Research in animal models dating to the 1940's showed that mice first infected with influenza virus developed severe pneumonia, when challenged a few days later by doses of bacteria. Studies of tissue obtained from the bronchial tree at autopsy suggest that epithelial lining of respiratory tissue damaged by viral infection allows enhanced adherence by bacteria capable of producing lethal infection.[94]

In 1900 a filter -passing agent was isolated from chickens with "fowl plague". It was not until 1955 that fowl plague was recognized as illness caused by type A influenza virus. In 1930 influenza A virus was first recovered from swine showing respiratory symptoms. A human source (throat washings) was used to infect an animal host(a ferret). Again the virus proved to be influenza A. Influenza B and C virus were identified between 1940 and 1950. The ability to propagate virus in chick embryo allantois sac formed the basis for extensive production of the influenza vaccine still used commercially today. In 1946 and 1947 the significance of widespread antigenic variation of the virus was recognized as vaccination failed to protect. The term "antigenic drift" was introduced in 1955 to indicate the shift in chemical composition of the antigenic protein molecule.[95] The mutation rate of influenza

---

93 McCullers, Jonathan A. "Preventing and Treating secondary Bacterial Infection with Antiviral Agents". *Antiviral Therapeutics*. vol.16 (2),2011, pp.123-135.

94 Petersdorf, R.G., Fusco, J.J, Harter, D.H. Albrink, W.S. "Pulmonary Infections complicating Asian Influenza". *AMA Archives Internal Medicine*. vol.103,1959, pp.262-272.

95 Koprowski, Hillary. *Microbe Hunters then and now*. Bloomington, Ill : Medi-Ed Press, 1996, p191.

virus and other RNA virus is rapid as is evolution in nature. Thus protection against this ever-changing infectious agent has remained a serious challenge throughout the century.

Viral hepatitis was known as" campaign jaundice "during various wars dating at least to the fifth century BC in Greece. Perhaps as many as 70,000 cases were recognized in Union troops during the American Civil War. An outbreak of hepatitis B was identified in 1883 during a small pox immunization program in Bremen, Germany. Of over 1,200 vaccinated workers 15% developed jaundice within several weeks to 8 months following inoculation. No jaundice was observed in several hundred unvaccinated employees. Not uncommonly the disease occurred in clinics for diabetes, venereal disease and tuberculosis. Infections were spread to those individuals during World War II as well as recipients of blood transfusions. The proximate cause of these misfortunes was at the time unrecognized as being related to contaminated needles syringes and serum. By 1955 serum enzyme assay provided evidence of hepatitis infection in individuals with or without jaundice.[96]

Viral hepatitis is an especially serious condition not only because of destruction of liver cells leading to cirrhosis but also the development of hepatocarcinoma. There is a hundred-fold increase incidence of cancer of the liver in chronic Hepatitis B carriers compared with non-carriers. Fortunately a highly effective vaccine has been developed against the virus. However the chronic carriers commonly succumb to their own immune response which leads to destruction of liver cells. Finally it must be noted that in addition to hepatitis B, HVA (hepatitis A) virus can be transmitted orally and shows a shorter incubation period. Other antigens (non A and non B) are designated hepatitis C--ultimately fatal if untreated.[97]

---

96 Koprowski, Hillary(*Microbe Hunters then and now*. Bloomington, Ill : Medi-Ed Press,1996, p214.

97 Koprowski, Hillary(1996)*Microbe Hunters then and now*. Bloomington, Ill Medi-Ed Press,1996, p217.

Chapter 9

Beyond Observation and Support: The Physician comes of Age

While historians may argue that the changes of the Roaring Twenties and 1930's including women's suffrage and prohibition were of paramount social importance, certain aspects of progress in medicine and Health Care during this period deserve our consideration. At the beginning of the twentieth century the number of. recognized legitimate medications available to the practicing physician were few in number. Primarily the list was limited to opioids (pain), aspirin (fever), anesthetics (ether, chloroform, cocaine), quinine(antimalarial), and digitalis derivatives(cardiac). It seems reasonable to suggest that the introduction of insulin in 1922 by Sir Frederick Banting and Charles Best produced the greatest *individual* compound bearing a life-saving impact during this period.[98] In 1901 Opie had shown that diabetes was attributable to destruction of the portion of the pancreas known as the Islets of Langerhans. Working in J.J.R. McLeod's laboratory in Toronto, Banting and Best isolated a purified protein preparation (later known as *insulin*) which they subsequently injected into a critically ill diabetic teenage boy thereby

---

98 Porter, Roy *The Greatest Benefit to Mankind*. New York, London: Horton and Company,1997, pp 567-8.

saving his life. Following this original case whole hospital wards of dying juvenile diabetics were similarly treated with this life-saving prescription yielding dramatic results in an otherwise fatal disease. These researchers were subsequently awarded the Nobel Prize in medicine.[99]

In 1849 Thomas Addison identified the severe impairment of adrenal gland function which has ever since born his name. This condition was superbly described by him in a paper entitled "On the constitutional topic and local effects of Diseases of the suprarenal capsules" in 1855. In a number of cases pathologic examination revealed tuberculous destruction of the adrenal cortex. Remarkably it was not until 1930 that W.W. Swingle and Pfeiffer were able to produce purified adrenal cortical extract.[100] Following their report in the journal "Science", Ball and Landsburg successfully treated a patient dying of Addison's Disease in 1930. By 1931 it had been shown that a lipid extract of adrenal cortical hormones could prolong indefinitely the life of adrenalectomized cats. Research carried out during the 1930's revealed the critical role of the adrenal cortex in conserving sodium in the body. Cortisone (Kendall's compound E) was prepared by Sarrett at Merck Laboratories in 1946 followed by the announcement that it would relieve symptoms of Rheumatoid Arthritis. Kendall himself won the Nobel Prize in 1950 for his research on corticosteroids. A second product of the adrenal gland "adrenaline" or epinephrine was discovered about 1920. Subsequent research identified nerve axons as conduits while actual transmission of impulses across synapses other nerves or to muscles or end organs was provided by chemicals acetylcholine, epinephrine and dopamine.

Major advances in neurology and neurosurgery were achieved during the interwar decades. In the 1920s Percival Bailey, a Northwestern University graduate became Cushing's assistant in

---

[99] Porter, Roy *The Greatest Benefit to Mankind*. New York, London: Horton and Company1997, p567.

[100] Swingle, W.W., and Pfeiffner, J.J., Am. J. Physiol; vol. 96 p153-156,1931

Boston where he painstakingly studied the brain tumors operated upon at the Peter Bent Brigham. By 1927 Bailey and Cushing had published an exhaustive formal classification of Gliomas.[101] Their studies differentiated between extremely malignant brain lesions designated "glioblastoma" which remain to this day fatal (within 1 to 2 years of diagnosis) and more benign tumors such as oligodendroglioma and cerebellar astrocytoma of childhood.[102] During these two decades Cushing also operated upon a group of truly benign lesions which he named "meningioma" since they arose from the brain coverings ("meninges") These tumors most often allow total resection and permanent cure. A famous exception to this concept was the case of General Leonard Wood on whom Cushing successfully operated prior to WW1. Wood held a successful command during World War I only to die from a recurrence of the previously operated meningioma about 20 years later.[103]

From a technical standpoint a major advance in the difficult problem concerning control of bleeding during cranial surgery was the introduction of an electro-surgical unit for cauterizing small arteries by W.T. Bovie in 1927. Cushing was able to report an accumulation of 780 verified cases of brain tumor by 1922, while Walter Dandy at Johns Hopkins had succeeded in *total* removal of a series of benign tumors designated acoustic neuroma. Meanwhile widespread advances in general medicine progressed slowly,

Improvement in the management of neurological problems should be noted following the founding in New York City of a Neurological Institute in 1909. By the end of World War I New York neurosurgeons had reported on hundreds of spinal operations. During the 1920s neurological surgery was being advanced at the Columbia

---

101 Bailey, P.C. and Cushing, H. *Tumors of the Glioma Group*. Philadelphia: J.P Lippincott, 1926.

102 Bailey Percival, Buchannan, Douglas and Bucy, Paul C. (*Intracranial Tumors of Infancy and of Childhood*, Chicago : University of Chicago Press,1948

103 Fulton, John Farquhar. *Harvey Cushing, a Biography* Springfield: Charles C.. Thomas, 1945.

Presbyterian hospital and later at the New York Hospital under Dr. Bronson Ray.[104] In 1926 important progress in neurological diagnosis was achieved when Egaz Moniz introduced the technique of cerebral angiography. Although this procedure for the **first time allowed detailed definition of the blood vessels of the brain by injection of contrast** material into an artery in the neck[105], full utilization did not occur for a number of years until the introduction of safer Iodinated contrast material. By 1937 neurologists had obtained a reliable anticonvulsant medication known as Dilantin which could control most epileptic seizures without producing the significant drowsiness which was frequently encountered with the administration of phenobarbital. One of the greatest achievements encompassing both medical and surgical progress during this period was the opening of the first true Blood Bank at the Cook County Hospital in Chicago in 1937. Although blood typing had been described in the early 20th century and the anticoagulant citrate was available during World War I, this was the first time that whole blood had been safely stored during extended periods for surgery and emergency treatment.[106]

During the 1930s physicians began to realize that children were not simply miniature adults. Having recognized the need for specialization in the treatment of neurological problems of infancy and childhood, Harvey Cushing assigned Franc Ingraham,[107] one of his brightest assistants, the task of developing the special area

---

104 Ray, Bronson S. M.D. "The Development of Neurosurgery in New York City". *Bulletin of the New YorAcademofMedicine*. Vol.55, No.10, November, 1979, pp916-936.

105 American College of Surgeons: *Remembering Milestones and achievements in Surgery* Tampa, Florida: Fairmount Media Group,2012, p123.

106 Giangrande, Paul I.F. "The History of Blood Transfusion". *British Journal of Hematology*,2000, vol.110 p758-767.

107 Cohen, Allen R., Vogel, Timothy W. and Hart, G.W. M.D. Ph.D., The Lost Art of Localization: Franc Ingraham's Legacy in Pediatric Neurosurgery. *J. Neurosurg. Pediatrics* 12, pp642-65, 2013.

of pediatric Neurosurgery.[108] Apart from the major problem of management of children with hydrocephalus, a number of conditions both medical and surgical are peculiar to this age group including congenital brain storage diseases, certain brain tumors, and subtypes of leukemia. Long term management of pediatric seizure disorders (epilepsy)was improved by Frederick Gibbs's development of EEG (electroencephalography). With this method he was not only able to confirm the presence of abnormal electrical brain activity but often the area of its origin. In 1938 definitive control of seizures in a large percentage of patients could be achieved following the introduction of Dilantin(Phenytoin). While several other drugs including Carbamazepine and phenobarbital are also available in the management of epilepsy, side effects may be distressing.[109]

Biochemical research improved treatment of children with significant developmental disorders e.g. celiac disease and phenylketonuria. Advances in spinal surgery allowed surgical closure of spina bifida and myelomeningocele in infants reducing not only mortality but often preventing severe disability.

In 1931 Jason Mixter and Joseph Barr at the Massachusetts General Hospital described what became the most widely diagnosed and surgically treated condition by almost all neurosurgeons: the herniated intervertebral disc. A review by Dr. Ernest Sachs of 900 laminectomies (spinal operations) over a 40 year period during the early 20th century yielded only 220 cases of herniated disc. Even more astonishing is the figure of 224 deaths–about one in four persons operated upon for a variety of spinal problems.[110] Based on personal experience of more than 1800 laminectomies performed since 1965 the postoperative mortality rate was far less than 1%. A best estimate

---

108 Fulton, John Farquhar. *Harvey Cushing, a Biography* Springfield: Thomas, Charles C.1945.

109) Merritt's Textbook of Neurology (7th edition) Ed. by Lewis P. Rowland M.D. (1984) Philadelphia: Lea and Febiger pp646-647.

110 Sachs, Ernest. "Some Observations based on a review of 900 laminectomies" *Bull. Of the New York Academy of Medicine*, 1950, pp370-377.

based on more than 30 years of practice is that busy neurosurgeons operated on 100-150 herniated discs per year in the lumbar and cervical spine. Prior to the 1930's individuals were often disabled by sciatica or arm pain from nerve root compression for months or years.

Concern regarding the role of streptococcal pharyngitis in the pathogenesis of rheumatic fever and endocarditis led to significant increase in the frequency of tonsillectomy by otolaryngologists. A study of 1000 children in New York City In 1934 revealed that two thirds of them (by age 11) had been subjected to tonsillectomy. After further assessment by panels of specialists all but 10 percent received a tonsillectomy.[111] Sadly a study performed in England at this time revealed that nearly 100 children per year died following tonsillectomy. Fortunately the introduction of antibiotics after WWII eliminated the need for tonsillectomy in the majority of children.

Concomitant with improved safety in anesthesia, ligation of a fetal blood vessel (patent ductus arteriosus) was carried out as a lifesaving measure by Dr Gross in Boston in 1938[112]. Following this procedure oxygenated blood from the lung could be returned to the infant's general circulation without mixing with unoxygenated "Blue" blood.

According to George Schambaugh, an outstanding otolaryngologist of the 20th century, an epochal advance in general medicine occurred in 1935 / 1936 with the introduction of Sulfonamides which had been synthesized in Germany about 1908. At the Rockefeller Institute in 1927 the compound had been added to quinine in order to increase antimalarial effectiveness. However it was not until 1927 that this sulfa drug was tested by Bayer researchers at the IG

---

111 Porter, Roy *The Greatest Benefit to Mankind*. New York, London: Horton and Company.1997, p601.

112 American College of Surgeons: *Remembering Milestones and achievements in Surgery*. Tampa, Florida : Fairmount Media Group, 2012, p100.

Farben Industries in Germany.[113] Although great success was initially achieved in the treatment of infections with "sulfa drugs", tragedy struck in 1937. In response to a demand for a better tasting product, the Massengill company's chief chemist designed a liquid consisting of sulfanilamide dissolved in ethylene glycol—a substance known by physicians to be toxic to the kidney. At least one hundred individuals (mainly children) were believed to have died as a result of this error before the product could be recalled. In 1938 Congress responded by passing the Pure Food, Drug and Cosmetic Act.

During the four decades following Lister's ground-breaking introduction of antiseptic surgery little had changed in the field of Orthopedics. Historically one should recall that several of Lister's earliest successes were cases of compound fractures of the extremities which prior to his discoveries would surely have required amputation to prevent infection and gangrene. In an outstanding review David Murray M.D. describes Orthopedics in 1913 as a specialty largely associated with "splints, straps and buckles "By the end of World War I bone grafting had been introduced by Dr. Fred Albee- in particular to stabilize tuberculous spines. 1925 Smith-Petersen described a three-prong nail for fixation of fractures of the femoral neck. Prior to this time hip fractures had been a catastrophic event for elderly people. Finally a suitable prosthesis for total replacement of the hip joint was introduced by Venable and Stuck (1936) and later improved by Smith- Petersen utilizing a vitallium cup. During this period the rehabilitation of disabled individuals including many victims of poliomyelitis were treated and benefited by orthopedic surgeons. Additional advances in Orthopedics were largely delayed until after World War II. [114]

---

113 Porter, Roy. *The Greatest Benefit to Mankind*. New York, London: Horton and Company,1997, p453.

114 American College of Surgeons: *Remembering Milestones and achievements in Surgery*. Tampa, Florida: Fairmount Media Group, 2012, pp132-137.

Chapter 10

Part 1: Pharmacology comes of age: Antibiotics and beyond

Those of us born in America during the Great Depression were scarcely aware of the horrors of war. While our daily lives were inconveniently touched by rationing of gasoline and a few foodstuffs, war was primarily something which we learned about in newspapers or heard described in a colorless radio broadcast. The two decades between my birth in 1936 and entrance into the Yale School of Medicine (1956) produced incredible geopolitical and scientific discoveries including the nuclear chain reaction (atomic bomb) and the structure of DNA. Meanwhile the availability of penicillin and alternative antibiotics for treatment of common bacterial infections during the 1940's contributed to a revolution in medical therapeutics comparable to Lister's introduction of antisepsis in surgery during the 1870s.

Prior to this time the physician's helplessness in the management of bacterial infection is clearly illustrated in reports documenting outbreaks of meningitis. In June 1905 Foster described a series of thirty cases in the New York epidemic. "It was long since noted that epidemics of meningitis occur in prisons and barracks where crowding is a feature and the slums of larger cities approach these conditions". He further describes the significant spread of infection within families.[115] Foster notes that "Osler records a family -five of whose members suffered from the disease and Serval reports six children in one family in the New York epidemic of 1872." A gram-negative diplococcus was found in the blood of these children by the pathologist W.J. Elser. Lumbar puncture showed Meningococcus in the spinal fluid. In two fatal cases lobar pneumonia had developed. In different epidemics the mortality from cerebrospinal meningitis varied from 28% to 75% with an average of 50%. Treatment of this devastating illness in the early 20th century consisted of darkening the room, an air mattress, and restraint of the patient. Further, copious administration of fluids along with opioid sedatives was recommended. Fortunately Thomas was able to record that "sulfadiazine was wonderfully effective" in the treatment of bacterial meningitis by 1941[116].

Lewis Thomas, who graduated from Harvard Medical School in 1937, notes that the "greater part of the work done on these (Boston City Hospital) wards was largely custodial". Patients did not report to the emergency room unless they feared for their life." The medicine which Thomas was trained to practice was essentially Osler's medicine."[117] It is worth recalling that Osler had been appointed Professor of Medicine at Hopkins in 1889.

In spite of the introduction of insulin (1923) a study of "contemporary medicine" in Malta found that very little progress had been made in controlling mortality for diabetics. Ventura's data indicate that the case specific mortality rose from 48/100,000 to 61/100,000 in 1938. The incidence of diabetics among the elderly was found to be 17% by 1961. As Porter points out such negative

---

115 Foster, N. B." Cerebrospinal meningitis: a study of thirty cases in the New York". *The American Journal of Medical Sciences (1827-1924)* June 1905.

116 Thomas, Lewis. *The Fragile Species*. New York: Collier Books, Macmillan Publishing Company, 1992 p75

117 Thomas, Lewis. *Medicine: The Youngest Science*. New York: The Viking Press, 1983, p28

data are primarily the result of increased prosperity and changing dietary habits.[118]

As preclinical medical students our introduction to modern pharmacology provided us with a sense that we were finally gaining basic knowledge regarding the tools which we would eventually apply in treating our patients. Throughout most of the 19th century the "Materia medica" was categorized into astringents, poultices, emetics, purgatives narcotics and laxatives. A system of therapeutics of the 19th century known as homeopathy was espoused by Hahnemann[119] based on the principle that in limited dosages "like cures like". Useful medicinal therapy in the early 20th century included polyvalent serum for infectious disease, digitalis, gold therapy for tuberculosis (doubtful value), morphine(and related opioids) for pain and the antimalarial quinine. One of the intern's primary tasks in the 1930's was identification of the specific type of pneumococcal organism causing pneumonia in the individual patient so that a specific antiserum could be produced and administered to the patient.[120]

Advances in organic chemistry and pharmacology provided a means to deal with two of Mankind's greatest known scourges. In addition to the dramatic effect of penicillin in treating syphilis, streptomycin had become available in 1943 as the first drug with effective action against tuberculosis. While TB was not considered universally fatal, it frequently passed through multiple generations of a family with resulting major disability-often later requiring complex surgery. It was during WWII that effective treatment of illness attributed to Streptococci, Staphylococci, Pneumococci, and Meningococci etc. was developed. These organisms, the culprits responsible for boils, abscesses, pneumonia, and meningitis, proved susceptible to

---

118 Porter, Roy (1997) The Greatest Benefit to Mankind. New York, London: Horton and Company p29,30

119 Porter, Roy. *The Greatest Benefit to Mankind*. New York, London: Horton and Company,1997, p390-391

120 Thomas, Lewis. *Medicine: The Youngest Science*. New York: The Viking Press,1983, p43,44

penicillin. Although Alexander Fleming had noted clearing of bacterial culture in dishes contaminated by penicillium mold as early as 1927, it was not until 1941 that the therapeutic value of Penicillin was appreciated by Drs. Chain and Fleury.[121] Syphilis had attacked human beings on a global scale for centuries. During pregnancy syphilitic mothers sustained miscarriage or produced stillborn infants. Congenital syphilis of infancy commonly resulted in severe rashes and bone abnormalities with eventual involvement of liver, spleen and brain. Adults were frequently unaware of infection until the rash of secondary syphilis appeared months later. Prior to the introduction of penicillin the only available treatment was Ehrlich's compound 606 known as Salvarsan.[122] Unfortunately the side effects of this arsenical compound limited its usefulness and general acceptability. If untreated, syphilis led to major widespread structural lesions in multiple organs. In the central nervous system it manifested either as a form of meningitis or a large tumorous structure known as a gumma. Fatality was the expected outcome of this tertiary stage of the disease usually many years after the initial infection. Prior to World War II an experimental study was undertaken at the Tuskegee Institute to longitudinally follow the course of the disease. By the time that penicillin had become available there was little if any doubt regarding the anticipated outcome. Tragically the curative drug[123] was withheld from these patients with predictable results.

By the 1950s introduction of antibiotics had focused attention of innumerable physicians on the management of acute infections including pharyngitis, tonsillitis, pneumonia and kidney infection which earlier had so frequently preceded fatal renal failure. These conditions could now often be controlled. The disabling and

---

121 Porter, Roy. *The Greatest Benefit to Mankind*. New York, London: Horton and Company 1997, pp456,457

122 Porter, Roy. *The Greatest Benefit to Mankind*. New York, London: Horton and Company, 1997, p452

123 Katzung, Bertram G. *Basic and Clinical Pharmacology*. Norwalk, Connecticut: Appleton and Lange,1995, p766

potentially fatal effects of meningitis particularly in childhood were largely preventable. During my years at the Yale School of Medicine (1956-1960) the management of infectious disease truly occupied center stage-undoubtedly related to the fact that the chairman of the Department of Medicine devoted his research activities to this area. I still recall that it was considered almost a sin to introduce a urinary catheter for fear of producing bacterial contamination and a urinary tract infection. However my own lifetime experience suggested that careful aseptic technique reduced the risk of this problem to a minimum. Several years later as a senior Neurosurgical resident at the George Washington University I experienced an interesting corollary to the concern regarding introduction of a foreign body into a patient. In this case an individual suffering from post-operative infection was being treated with intravenous antibiotics. Infection persisted until the IV needle and tubing had been removed and replaced with a new apparatus. Following further study it was determined that bacteria had colonized the intravenous tubing.

Physicians could be optimistic by the early 1960s in regard to the virtual elimination of certain surgical procedures. No longer was amputation or disfigurement / disability likely to be the outcome of osteomyelitis. Brain abscess was almost completely eliminated following cases of meningitis or septicemia. The majority of pulmonary infections rarely evolved into lung abscess or empyema requiring surgical drainage. Unfortunately many viral illnesses including encephalitis, hepatitis, pneumonia and AIDS remained as major medical problems which required further research.

The advent of psychopharmacology[124] eliminated the need for the semi-barbaric procedure known as "lobotomy". As recently as 1950 a film was produced in Hollywood entitled "The Snake Pit" which referred to an ancient form of therapy for mentally disturbed individuals. Prior to the introduction of phenothiazine compounds (e.g. Thorazine) psychotic patients had been treated with straight-

---

124 Katzung, Bertram G. *Basic and Clinical Pharmacology*. Norwalk, Connecticut: Appleton and Lange,1995, p432,437-8

jackets, ice baths and electroshock therapy. If that failed, the most severely disturbed were subjected to destructive brain surgery (prefrontal lobotomy) which rendered them docile but intellectually disabled. During the following decade a major neuro-active drug (L-dopa) was introduced to treat Parkinson's disease, characterized by involuntary shaking and lethargy. The drug was found to act as a replacement for dopamine, a natural neurotransmitter secreted by the human substantia nigra.[125]

A major breakthrough in the medical treatment of a common mental disorder occurred when imipramine (Tofranil), the first tricyclic antidepressant, was introduced in 1962.[126] Dr. Freyhan (University of Pennsylvania) reported 30% optimal results in a group of patients diagnosed as" depressive psychosis" describing failure in 20%. The drug was found to have significant effect on the blockage of Serotonin and norepinephrine reuptake. Unfortunately the medication is contraindicated in patients suffering from schizophrenia. The Introduction of one tranquilizer ended in tragedy. Around 1960 in England administration of Thalidomide (prescribed to reduce "morning sickness" of pregnancy) produced severe genetic defects in the developing fetus.[127] The children were born, either without limbs or with flipper-like appendages. Outstanding work by Dr. Frances Kelsey at the University of Chicago prevented the FDA from releasing this drug in the United States.

---

125 Katzung, Bertram G. *Basic and Clinical Pharmacology*. Norwalk, Connecticut : Appleton and Lange,1995, p420-421

126 Katzung, Bertram G. *Basic and Clinical Pharmacology*. Norwalk, Connecticut: Appleton and Lange1995, p453

127 Katzung, Bertram G. *Basic and Clinical Pharmacology*. Norwalk, Connecticut: Appleton and Lange,1995, p 914

Chapter 10

Part 2

Those of us fortunate enough to graduate from medical school in the 1960s were now equipped with a wide range of therapeutic options which seem to grow exponentially. During the ensuing decade bacterial penicillinase-resistant antibiotics became available to treat skin, respiratory, and bone infections. Invasion by the more challenging coliform and enteric organisms was usually susceptible to Gentamicin and Chloramphenicol. To be sure certain organisms proved resistant and challenging-often related to antibiotics previously prescribed for the patient's less acute health problems. Prophylactic administration of antibiotics prior to surgery was able to reduce the rate of infection in clean areas such as the central nervous system to almost zero. The treatment of burns with sulfa compounds applied to the skin allowed regeneration and decreased infection in the areas requiring grafting. An improved understanding of the role of hypertension led to a reduction in the frequency of stroke and cerebrovascular disease. In general the control of blood pressure could frequently be achieved by a combination of reduced salt diet and newly formulated thiazide diuretics.[128] Prior to the 1960's fluid reduction in congestive heart

---

128 Katzung, Bertram G. *Basic and Clinical Pharmacology*. Norwalk, Connecticut : Appleton and Lange,1995, pp239-241

failure and hypertension was achieved by treatment with Thiomerin a Mercury-containing diuretic with known toxicity.[129] Drugs which blocked the sympathetic nervous system including Inderal and methyldopa provided additional improvement in the control of blood pressure.. Advances in radiologic diagnosis and anticoagulant therapy added prophylaxis against clotting in major vessels serving the brain and heart. During the early 1960s the role of nicotine and combustion products in smoke had been identified as major factors in respiratory disease and lung cancer. Reduction in smoke inhalation not only decreased the incidence of chronic bronchitis and emphysema but also reduced the deleterious effects of nicotine on blood vessels which had contributed to hypertension.

Pharmacology clearly played an important role in the management of coma and semi-comatose states. In 1964 most patients brought to the DC General Hospital (where I was assigned as a neurosurgical resident) in a state of impaired consciousness came under our care. It was urgent that we determine whether the patient's condition was secondary to. a head injury, brain tumor, cerebrovascular accident or metabolic disturbance such as diabetes or ingestion of a toxic substance. Our frequent approach to the problem was the injection of contrast material which could safely demonstrate the size and position of cerebral. blood vessels on x-ray With this information one could demonstrate the blockage of an artery as the cause of a stroke or displacement of vessels by a tumor mass or a blood clot pressing on the brain surface. An additional diagnostic tool available at this time was the "brain scan". Images were obtained following the injection of a radiopharmaceutical such as technetium. This technique provided an essentially risk-free method of localization of certain mass cerebral lesions. Additionally, we now had significant medical means to

---

129 Stewart, Harold J, M.D., McCoy, Herbert I., M.D., Shepard, Edward M., M.D. and Luckey, E. Hugh, M.D. "Experience with Thiomerin a New Mercurial Diuretic" *Circulation*,1950, pp502-507

temporarily control intracranial pressure utilizing osmotic diuretics (mannitol and urea) and corticosteroids given intravenously. These drugs proved to be of great advantage in preventing disability or death both pre and postoperatively.

Chapter 11

Surgical surprises-encounters with unexpected pathology

By the 1960s there was rarely if ever any doubt in regard to size and location of space occupying pathology involving the nervous system. While anecdotal experiences rarely have provided major improvement in patient care, a description of unexpected findings encountered at operation may prove of interest for the reader. While a resident at the Children's Hospital of Washington, D.C., I assisted a neurosurgeon who was performing a brain biopsy at the request of a medical neurologist. In this case we were dealing with a severely brain impaired infant whose condition could not be explained. It should be recalled that we did not have the luxury of CT scanning or MRI at that time. Upon exposing the surface of the cerebral cortex we encountered a covering which had the appearance of greenish tar. I have never seen anything close to this appearance since that moment. Sadly the child's brain was encased by malignant melanoma which had arisen from the arachnoid(covering) layer of cells.

Later that same year, as chief resident at the VA Hospital in Washington DC, we operated upon a gentleman with a markedly swollen but firm temporal area of the skull. While benign tumors (meningioma) are commonly found in this location the diagnosis in this case was Hodgkin's Disease- a form of lymphoid malignancy. A few years later evidence accumulated that such tumors were not un- commonly encountered in patients infected with HIV.

On another occasion in 1965 Dr. Watts had operated upon a young man for malignant tumor of the frontal lobe of the brain. Initially the patient appeared to be making a good recovery until he presented at follow up with a large mass in his cheek. Apparently the brain tumor had escaped the skull and implanted in the facial soft tissues He was initially able to obtain some relief through radiation therapy but eventually succumbed to the malignant glioma.

As an attending surgeon at the National Hospital for Orthopedics and Rehabilitation in Arlington, Virginia I often worked with an orthopedist when spinal fusion was planned. On one such occasion the lumbar paravertebral muscle was exposed and elevated from the spine producing an inordinate amount of venous bleeding. After satisfactory control of the hemorrhage we found the source to be multiple small pale tumors attached to the undersurface of the muscle which had arisen from a previously undetected malignancy.

Several operations to be described produced unexpected positive results. During my year at the DC General Hospital a young man with weakness of one side of his body was found to have a positive technetium brain scan. After confirmation with arteriography he was operated upon. A large needle was passed into the mass which allowed evacuation of old liquefied brain hemorrhage. The patient made a rapid recovery of limb movement in a case in which preoperatively a malignant tumor had been suspected.

In 1967 at the VA Hospital a patient came to us with severe quadriplegia. He had not sustained a spinal injury but was found to have a large mass at the base of the brain. At surgery a huge thrombosed aneurysm (swollen artery) was found to be compressing the brain stem. Excision of the mass produced a dramatic resolution of his motor weakness.

As a neurosurgeon on active duty with the USAF I encountered a number of challenging problems. It was axiomatic that persistent leakage of spinal fluid from the nose or ear required surgical intervention to prevent meningitis. In one particular case I found several openings in the skull base underlying the brain- the result of a gunshot wound. Once visualized, it was efficient to literally "caulk" the apertures with methyl methacrylate which we had frequently used to provide closure of cranial vault defects.

A particularly gratifying experience was the treatment of a young man who had developed marked increased intracranial pressure which was obvious on examining his eyes. Ventriculography showed a blockage of the spinal fluid from the fourth ventricle at the base of the brain. At operation a tumor mass was identified within the fourth ventricle. I was able to detach the mass from the brainstem and restore fluid passage. The patient was given radiation therapy to the area and survived many years in excellent health. I subsequently received a Christmas card from him and his wife for many years.

After I had been in practice for about ten years an individual with severe weakness in his arms and legs was brought to the emergency department. While awaiting the results of several tests the patient decided to leave the hospital. Fortunately, following identification of the problem, the Emergency Room Physicians were able find and return him to the hospital for treatment. After confirmation of his problem by a myelogram, he was operated upon. Much to my surprise surgery disclosed an abscess which was compressing the spinal cord-most likely related to his long standing intravenous drug use. For many weeks the patient remained quadriplegic, but one morning he showed me that he could wiggle his toes. I was incredulous at first but he slowly recovered. About 18 months later I found him walking down a hospital corridor aided only by a single short arm crutch. That was surely the most remarkable recovery from a severe spinal cord lesion which I'd ever encountered.

In 1967, shortly before completion of my tour in the USAF, a young man was sent to us having survived a self-inflicted gunshot wound of the right side of his skull. Both the patient and the Air Force were anxious for a cosmetic restoration. The patient had excellent speech and cognition but definite impairment of a left-sided motor function in his extremities. Initially I planned simply to restore his skull to its natural convex shape. However after elevation of the scalp, marked scarring with adhesions to the brain surface were encountered. This scar tissue was dissected meticulously from the brain surface and the whole area was covered with a synthetic patch. The skull defect which measured around 10 centimeters by 10 centimeters was filled with methyl methacrylate. The patient made a rapid recovery which included restoration of the use of his left extremities. The dramatic recovery of motor function was truly unpredicted.

Chapter 12

Part 1: Tuberculosis and the emergence of thoracic surgery

However tempting to consider advances and success in public health as "case closed", prevention of epidemic recurrence requires ongoing vigilance. One might optimistically assume that the enormous mortality from bubonic and pneumonic plague during the 14th century in Europe would have permanently eradicated this disease. Unfortunately plague, although seemingly dormant, erupted in Eastern Europe in the Black Sea and Crimean area with a vengeance during the 19th century. It was finally brought under control by intensive quarantine measures enforced in Odessa, Ukraine by Richelieu, an officer in the czar's army.

Mortality statistics during the first half of the 20th century were published by Grove and Hetzel for the United States department of health education and Welfare in 1968.[130] A few statistics from this exhaustive treatise appear worth consideration.

Listed below are leading causes of deaths per 100,000 population in the United States:

---

[130] Grove, Robert D. Ph.D. and Hetzel, Alice M. *Vital Statistic Rates in the United States 1940-1960*. United States dept. of Health Education and Welfare, Washington D.C., 1968

Year.	Disease.	Number per 100 K population
1900	1) pneumonia	200
	2) Tuberculosis	198
	3) Heart disease	145
	4) Stroke	105
1960	1) heart disease	350
	2) Cancer	150
	3) Stroke	140

The introduction of antibiotics and major Innovative Public Health measures produced a significant reduction in infectious pulmonary disease just as the discovery of insulin had done for control of diabetes. The death rate for syphilis and tuberculosis was reduced to 2 and 1.5 per 100,000 people respectively. When one considers the statistical significance of these mortality data it is incumbent upon the reader to recall that the white population of the entire United States was limited to 76 million persons in 1900. Thus about 144,000 deaths from T.B. occurred in the entire country from this group. By 1960 the population of the United States had grown to 180 million with accidents occupying the fourth position in mortality of 74/100 thousand for males.

The Vital Statistics department of HEW list Tuberculosis as the second leading cause of death in the United States.[131] This disease had declined to number 6 by 1930 and is no longer listed among the top 10 causes of death by 1960. In order to control the spread of tuberculosis in the general population several significant Public

---

131 Grove, Robert D. Ph.D. and Hetzel, Alice M. *Vital Statistic Rates in the United* States 1940-1960. United States dept. of Health Education and Welfare, Washington D.C., 1968

Health measures were introduced. The most important of these was the tuberculosis sanitarium. An article published in the Chicago Tribune 1909 described TB as the city's "worst problem". In an effort to deal with this situation a sanitarium had been opened in the Chicago suburb of Naperville in 1907. I had the opportunity to work with Dr. Jerome Head for several months as a surgical resident in 1961. Dr. Head had been the chief medical officer of this TB facility between 1949 and 1955 when it had been converted to a General Hospital. Several of the former patients was still being cared for at the Northwestern University's Chicago Wesley Memorial Hospital since their condition remained precarious.

Gilberto Gonzalez MD described the year 1961 to 1962 spent in the MTS (Municipal Tuberculosis Sanitarium of Chicago) as a resident surgeon. He pointed out that many of the patients had previously been confined for years in sanitaria. Detention in many cases was not unlike patients with mental disease. Although Streptomycin introduced after World War II alleviated the problem, a major leap forward in the medical control of tuberculosis occurred with the introduction of Rifampin during the 1960s.

The development of lung surgery in the United Kingdom is superbly described by Smith.[132] Apparently a few Isolated efforts at partial lung removal had been recorded by the beginning of the 20th century. The fear of collapse of the lung when pneumothorax occurred was the great inhibitory influence hindering the development of thoracic surgery. At the Brampton hospital 13 operations were carried out for empyema in an effort to remove infectious material from inside the chest. During the first quarter of the century an apparatus was designed to maintain positive pressure within the lung in an effort to prevent collapse. While the fear of collapse of the lung during chest surgery remained problematic, partial limited *collapse therapy* remained the best hope for a successful surgical treatment of tuberculosis until 1948. Unfortunately 70% of patients (3500 total

---

132 Smith, R. Abbey. "Development of lung surgery in the United Kingdom". *Thorax*, vol. 37,1982, pp161-168

cases) treated in 1926 had eventually died. The surgical treatment required partial removal of multiple ribs with resulting chest deformities and marked reduction in breathing capacity. During the 1920 to 1930 period a number of operations were carried out for bronchiectasis(an intrapleural infectious process) with limited success. Utilizing a method observed in Toronto Canada 10 patients operated upon for bronchiectasis yielded a bronchopleural fistula rate of 50%. However hospital mortality was reduced from 50% to 20%. In 1933 Evarts Graham in the United States performed the first successful pneumonectomy for carcinoma of the lung.[133] The control of bronchopleural fistula by improved surgical techniques combined with antibiotic therapy after 1944 represented the major reduction in postoperative morbidity and mortality. During the 1950s. advanced nursing care, physiotherapy, endotracheal suctioning and positive pressure ventilation all contributed to far better results from thoracic surgery. By 1939. Edwin Churchill MD. of the Massachusetts General Hospital was able to perform segmental lung resection.[134]

Dr. Maxwell Chamberlain, a 1933 graduate of University of Kansas; completed his surgical training in Ann Arbor in 1938 following which he practiced as a thoracic surgeon for New York State. Following Military service he became internationally famous for the technique of segmental pulmonary resection.

Major advances in the field of pulmonary pathology and physiology were made by the research of A.A. Liebow, a 1935 graduate of the Yale school of Medicine. Dr. Liebow devoted his entire career to the anatomy of the human lung--especially to the relationship between the airways and the vasculature which exchange and transport blood gases. Detailed understanding of pulmonary structure promoted

---

[133] American College of Surgeons. *Remembering Milestones and achievements in Surgery*. Tampa, Florida : Fairmount Media Group, 2012, p100

[134] American College of Surgeons. *Remembering Milestones and achievements in Surgery*. Tampa, Florida : Fairmount Media Group,2012

major advances in pulmonary surgery during the next two decades. Lindskog states that mortality following thoracic trauma decreased dramatically from about. 90% in 1900 to 50%after WW1 to 10% following WWII.[135]

---

[135] Lindskog, Gustave E. M.D. "Averill Abraham Liebow (1911-1978) A Colleague's Tribute". *The Yale Journal of Biology and Medicine,* vol.54, 1981, pp127-137

CHAPTER 12

Part 2: Dawn of cardiovascular surgery

A number of articles reviewing this area attribute the ligation of a blood vessel linking the aorta and pulmonary artery (ductus arteriosus) by Dr. Gross in 1938 as the first planned vascular procedure in the chest.[136] This relatively simple but previously untested surgery allowed the infant's brain and body to receive fully oxygenated blood for the first time. Incredibly the surgeon's chief forbade him to repeat the procedure on a second deserving child. Finally in 1944 Alfred Blalock at Johns Hopkins hospital successfully operated upon a child whose diagnosis by pediatrician Helen Tausig was "Tetralogy of Fallot. "a cardiovascular problem which also markedly reduced oxygenated blood flowing away from the heart. Blaylock's successful procedure has been immortalized as the "blue baby" 0peration.[137]

During WWII military surgeons such as Dwight Harken recognized the need for a technique which allowed successful entry into the human heart to permit removal of bullet and shell fragments. Following a series of experimental operations on dogs a procedure

---

136 American College of Surgeons. *Remembering Milestones and achievements in Surgery*. Tampa, Florida: Fairmount Media Group, 2012, p100

137 American College of Surgeons. *Remembering Milestones and achievements in Surgery*. Tampa, Florida: Fairmount Media Group, 2012, p100

was developed which could be used in human surgery. By 1948 Charles Bailey of Philadelphia had reported on an operation which permitted the surgeon entry to the beating heart in order to relieve mitral stenosis, an obstruction of this orifice which led to heart failure and death. By 1952 Lillehei at the University of Minnesota had utilized a procedure which employed induced hypothermia. Prior to surgery the patient, a five year old girl, was cooled to 81 degrees allowing the surgeons time to safely enter her heart and close a septal defect. During the 1960s a similar technique was employed by neurosurgeons to allow safer surgery on cerebral aneurysms.[138]

In 1953 Dr. Michael DeBakey of Houston introduced the technique of endarterectomy--a quantum leap both in arterial surgery and prophylaxis against stroke. Prior to this time anticoagulation was the only available therapy for the prevention and or treatment of cerebral vascular disease. As noted in a previous chapter the narrowing of arteries carrying blood to the brain could be detected through arteriography. Thus one could now demonstrate radiographically the exact location of narrowing or clot in an artery–a problem which now could be attacked surgically. At last a method of reducing the frequency and severity of a stroke was available for a portion of the population. By the 1960s (when I graduated. from Medical School) the operation known as carotid endarterectomy was being performed frequently in large medical centers. As the surgical acumen improved for dealing with arteries, research progressed in technology for operating directly on the heart itself.

Probably the most important contribution to the surgeon's ability to perform extended open--heart procedures e.g. the replacement of damaged valves was the heart-lung machine. During the late 1950s a device commonly referred to as a'" bubble oxygenator" allowed the patient's entire circulation to bypass the heart permitting safe surgery in a clean dry field.[139] Speaking from experience as a very

---

[138] Pioneers of heart surgery NOVA official website 04.08.97

[139] American College of Surgeons. *Remembering Milestones and achievements in Surgery* Tampa, Florida : Fairmount Media Group, 2012, p100-101.

young assistant in 1961, the most time-consuming portion of the operation was attachment of the patient's large blood vessels to the machine prior to opening the heart. One could then proceed to excise the damaged heart valve and replace it with a new synthetic device. In. 1969 Dr. Denton Cooley performed the first human heart transplant in the USA allowing the patient a few extra months of life. Unfortunately the procedure has many limitations including rejection of the donor heart. A 2016 obituary of Dr. Cooley described a female patient who is currently living and well 30 years after a successful heart transplant.

Following World War II advances in vascular surgery allowed development of a technique for bypassing the liver known as a portacaval shunt in patients with advanced cirrhosis of the liver due to infectious hepatitis or alcoholism. In cirrhotic patients blood cannot pass normally through this organ leading to impairment of venous flow from the intestinal tract with subsequent accumulation of fluid(ascites) in the abdomen. Although the procedure was not a cure for cirrhosis it does reduce the severe accumulation of fluid in the peritoneal cavity and abdominal organs. Although originally a major open surgical procedure, these shunts can now be performed percutaneously by a radiologist.

Chapter 13

Part 1: Hospitals and training

A report of statistics from the Department of Virginia following the American Civil War indicates that of 293 thousand hospital admissions almost 20 thousand died.[140] Obviously many more deaths occurred among soldiers not evacuated promptly from the battlefields. Among those hospitalized were included 6,000 cases of measles, 3545 men with syphilis and 4500 infected with gonorrhea.[141] As was discussed in an earlier chapter an understanding of the mechanism of infectious disease and antisepsis was simply not available to the dedicated surgeons, nurses and auxiliary hospital personnel who attempted to save the sick and wounded. From a practical standpoint the problem of widespread dissemination of information regarding acceptable healthcare standards remained unsolved prior to WW1. A major effort to alleviate suffering of the sick and wounded was initiated in 1861 by formation of The Sanitary Commission which began as an all-purpose welfare agency in New York. Developed as a charitable organization by volunteers, its goal was to provide clothing,

---

140 Denney, Robert. *Civil War Medicine: Care and Comfort of the Wounded*. New York: Sterling Publishing Co.,1994, p11.

141 Denney, Robert. *Civil War Medicine: Care and Comfort of the Wounded*. New York: Sterling Publishing Co.,1994, p 66.

blankets, bandages and food for the casualties of war.[142] A fundamental problem encountered by medical personnel was that of transport ".. following the battle of Manassas as many as 7627 Confederate wounded were transported by train to a hospital in Gordonsville, VA. Large numbers died during transport". The wounded lay all night at the depot without care. Frederick Law Olmsted [143] described the important use of steamships by the Commission to transfer Union wounded by sea from Virginia to New York and Boston. To this end volunteers secured the steamship "Daniel Webster" which they cleaned exhaustively to create a hospital atmosphere--in the process avoiding cost to the government.

Following are several case histories as described in "United States Sanitary Commission Memoirs": Case XXIII: Axillary Artery severed by gunshot projectile: Hemorrhage not troublesome; consecutive gangrene of arm. A ball had penetrated left shoulder from behind. No radial pulse. Four days after wounding left arm became dark and swollen. Pt died on June 6.

Case LIV: Intermediary hemorrhage from a stump on the 14th day after amputation. Gunshot fracture of left humerus. May18,1864 AMPUTATION of left arm between middle and superior third. Admitted to Stanton Hospital May 21. On May 23d profuse arterial hemorrhage. Wound opened and artery secured. May 27 purulent matter discharged. May 29 and 30 pyogenic chills. June 4 pyogenic pneumonia. DIED same day. A surgeon noted that "almost every case of secondary amputation performed in Stanton Hospital during May and June 1864 proved fatal."

Significant progress in health care delivery was achieved on the East Coast(USA) at the Massachusetts General Hospital, Bellevue Hospital and Philadelphia General Hospital during the second half of the 19th century. The facilities in New York were of particular

---

142 Denney, Robert. *Civil War Medicine: Care and Comfort of the Wounded* New York: Sterling Publishing Co.,1994, pp18-19.

143 Denney, Robert. *Civil War Medicine: Care and Comfort of the Wounded*. New York: Sterling Publishing Co.,1994, p28.

importance in dealing with the millions of immigrants fleeing Russia and Eastern Europe, often accompanied by serious threats to Public Health such as tuberculosis.

The development of medical care in a major city further West can be illustrated by events in Chicago. Shortly before the American Civil War the physicians of Rush Medical College opened a twelve bed facility in the "downtown" area at Rush and North Water Streets. Patients were charged $3.00 per week! In 1851 the supervisors of Cook County asked the Sisters of Mercy to provide nursing care--subsequently transferring control to the Order. Mercy Hospital remains the longest running hospital facility in the city to this day. In 1863 the hospital relocated from the Chicago Loop to the near South Side and affiliated with what eventually became Northwestern University's medical school. Numerous hospital facilities were founded during the late 1800's by religious groups including Catholics, Jews, Lutherans, Methodists, and Baptists. Specialty hospitals began to appear during the last quarter of the 19th century. Noteworthy was the Chicago Lying in Hospital founded in 1895 by Joseph B. DeLee in a tenement house. By 1930 a massive building bearing De Lee's name had become part of the University of Chicago's medical center on 59th street. With the advent of health insurance in the 1930's a dramatic increase in hospital expansion and construction occurred. Although the original 971 bed Cook County Hospital had been completed in 1917 its continued expansion reached around 3000 beds by mid-century. Michael Reese, a South Side "private" hospital, opened to all races and religions in 1880. The original building was replaced by a 1000 bed facility in 1907. Although economic and physical decline of the neighborhood had begun in the 1940's, the hospital purchased adjacent properties and added additional clinics. It finally closed in 2008 after a merger. The property is under consideration for re-development by Amazon.

At the time of WWI, Ernest Codman, a surgeon on staff at the Massachusetts General Hospital stated "Every hospital should follow every patient it treats long enough to determine whether or not the treatment has been successful".[144] Due to inadequate hospital records (prior to the 20th century) it was difficult for physician applicants to fulfill requirements for admission to the American College of Surgeons. In addition to limited record keeping, many hospitals lacked minimal laboratory and radiologic services. In 1917 the ACS formulated "The Minimum Standard"[145] a document which required organized hospital staffs, governing policies and staff meetings to review the work of various departments including results of treatment. The Minimum Standard also required detailed record keeping, maintenance of laboratory facilities and an X-ray department. A survey in 1913 found that only 12% of 692 hospitals met the standard. By 1923 80% of hospitals having more than 100 beds had complied. The ACS became the sole executor of the hospital standardization process between 1918 and 1951. Responsibility for this process was assumed by the "Joint Commission on Accreditation of Hospitals" after 1951. The latter consisted of representatives of the AMA, ACS, and the American Hospital Association.

The most obvious defect attributable to military field hospitals prior to the twentieth century lay in failure to secure a continuous supply of uncontaminated water. Construction of buildings whose water supply did not depend on wells or creeks adjacent to latrines (or trenches) proved fundamental to the reduction of hospital mortality from dysentery and typhoid.

---

144 American College of Surgeons. *Remembering Milestones and achievements in Surgery*. Tampa, Florida: Fairmount Media Group, 2012, p67.

145 American College of Surgeons. *Remembering Milestones and achievements in Surgery*. Tampa, Florida: Fairmount Media group, 2012, p69.

Chapter 13

Part 2: Hospitals and Training

    Very little reference has previously been made in this book in regard to the major role of nurses whose contribution to modern medical care is of paramount importance. Formal training of nursing students did not begin in the United States until 1872. During the American Civil War a variety of dedicated individuals, both male and female, most with little or no experience provided essential care for the sick and wounded. Although microbes had not yet been identified with certainty for their role in disease and infection, many basic concepts of hygiene and nutrition were practiced whenever possible by nursing personnel. In the 1850's Florence Nightingale had arrived at the barracks hospital of Scutari (Turkey)[146] where she discovered filthy, malodorous rooms, infested by vermin and rodents. She and her staff launched a campaign of intense cleaning and scrubbing of the entire facility combined with adequate ventilation. Similar concepts were introduced by the U.S. Sanitary commission whose nurses included Clara Barton. Additionally, considerable effort was made to provide the patients with adequate nutrition although understanding of the role of vitamins still lay in the future.

---

146 Torvald, Jürgen. *The Century of The Surgeon*. New York: Pantheon Books Inc.,1957, p169-179.

Linda Richards described her first experience as a nursing pupil in 1872 at the New England Hospital for Women and children Roxbury, Massachusetts.[147] The program was organized by Dr. Susan Dimock who had completed four years of medical training in Europe. The facility served sixty patients and began with five student nurses, four interns and a resident physician. As each ward of six patients emptied the area was thoroughly scrubbed prior to re-use. Having completed her training, Ms. Richards was offered a position–first at the Belleview Hospital (New York) Training School. After a year she transferred to Boston to manage the teaching program for nurses at the Massachusetts General Hospital. The then current practice applicable to dealing with a typhoid patient required that every article used by him is kept separate in a special place. Articles which will not be injured are kept in a 2% solution of formaldehyde. All bed linen and articles are disinfected by the same solution. Dishes, trays and glasses are boiled immediately after use. During the early twentieth century Typhoid was essentially conceded to be a nursing problem. In considerable detail attention is given to the process of feeding, bathing and administering fluid via intramuscular or subcutaneous injection to patients too ill to have fluid by mouth. In reference to pneumonia cases all treatment and nursing care are directed to preventing cardiac failure and helping the patient through the period of toxemia. Avoiding constipation was also felt to be of significance.

During the first half of the 20th century certain procedures including insertion of intravenous needles, urinary catheters and administration of blood transfusions were assigned to Interns (first year after M.D.). At the Grace–New Haven Hospital these physicians received room and board supplemented by $25.00 per month wage as recently as 1960. Interns worked daily for 36 of each 48 hours in addition to full-time on alternate weekends. A major advance in patient care was achieved by introduction of "Intensive care Units" for serious postoperative neurosurgical and thoracic surgical cases.

---

147 Richards, Linda. "Early Days in the first American Training School for Nurses." *The American Journal of Nursing* vol.16, No. 3, Dec.1915, pp.174-179.

These units also undertook responsibility for care of individuals who had sustained major trauma. The Maryland Institute for Emergency Medical Services was opened in 1968 in Baltimore.

In accordance with the wishes of Johns Hopkins (d.1873), certificates of incorporation for a hospital and a university were filed in 1867.[148] Considered an expert on hospital construction, based in part on his Civil War experience, John Shaw Billings was invited to join the Hopkins Committee on hospital construction. As a member of the U.S. Surgeon General's team he had published circulars on barracks and hospitals as well as "a Report on the Hygiene of the United States Army". Billings felt that the hospital aims were not only to look after the sick poor but also "to promote discoveries in the science and art of medicine…and provide the means of giving medical instruction". Billings offered a plan for the physical design of the hospital based on his experience during the Civil War and inspection of many U.S. Marine Hospitals. The final plan for the Johns Hopkins Hospital was adopted by the Board of Trustees in 1876. The fully constructed facility did not open until 1889; fourteen years after Daniel Gilman had become president of the newly opened University. Four years later (1893) the School of Medicine opened under the tutelage of professors Welch, Osler, Halsted and Kelly. As the twentieth century progressed, university departments of Medicine essentially became bound to teaching hospitals. Training of 3d and 4th year medical students was for the most part achieved through physicians employed by the university ensuring control of the curriculum. These hospitals were staffed by resident physicians-in-training who also played a fundamental role in teaching medical students.

In contrast to increased privatization in the United States the British Government began to assume control of healthcare prior to WWll. These measures proved especially effective in dealing

---

148 Chapman, Carleton B. *Order out of Chaos*, Boston: Science History Publications, 1992. p108-110.

with victims of the "Blitz". In 1948 under a Labor Government the publicly funded NHS (National Health Service) was launched.[149]

The system provided *free* healthcare to legal residents at the point of service--funded through general taxation. Personal observation during a year in London and more recent video depiction indicated that a majority of patients were treated in a "ward" setting. Although there was initial resistance, the general physicians are now employed by the NHS. In contrast most physicians in the US have remained self-employed or under contract to large hospital corporations.

---

149 Porter, Roy. *The Greatest Benefit to Mankind*. New York, London: Horton and Company, 1997, p653.

Chapter 13

Part 3

In the following paragraphs an effort will be made to compare the physician's training and hospital care available in mid-twentieth century with the situation around 1900. My personal experience with hospitals spans a 67 year period from 1941 to 2007 both from the standpoint of patient and as a caregiver. By 1941 the business of hospital medicine had dramatically expanded. As a small boy I was treated at the Chicago Wesley Memorial Hospital, a brand new 21 story facility in downtown Chicago's "Gold Coast". Shortly thereafter "Chicago Wesley" became the premier teaching facility for the Northwestern University School of Medicine. Three years later I endured a tonsillectomy at the Johns Hopkins Hospital in Baltimore. During the next few years antibiotics (and good fortune) kept me from the hospital until 1958 when I began assisting in patient care while a medical student at Yale. For the first time I was exposed to many individuals with serious illness–whose care was primarily the responsibility of dedicated trained nurses and resident physicians who were 2-5 years beyond medical school.

Following my graduation (1960) I returned to Chicago Wesley Memorial as an intern which took me through rotations assisting in the care of patients on the services of medicine, surgery, obstetrics and pediatrics. It was then that I obtained a license to practice medicine and surgery independently i.e. without formal supervision. Following a year of residency in general surgery, a Fellowship provided by the International College of Surgeons enabled me to spend year training in neurology and neuropathology at The National Hospitals for Nervous Diseases in London in preparation for a career in neurological surgery.

During the period July 1963-64 I served as an assistant resident in neurosurgery under Dr. Paul C. Bucy renown for his research on the motor cortex of the brain. During that year my time was mainly spent performing cerebral arteriograms and examining patients. In June, 1964 I began three years of training in neurological surgery under Professor James W. Watts at George Washington University. My first year in Washington represented a dramatic contrast with almost all my previous medical training. At the D.C. General Hospital I was immersed in a plethora of neurological emergencies as assistant to Chief Resident Hamid Gokalp who was soon to become an outstanding neurosurgeon in Turkey. During that year we dealt with head injuries, cerebral hematomas, gunshot wounds and brain tumors as well as various spinal conditions. Not infrequently it was necessary to wheel our patients from the huge emergency department to our neuro unit somewhat reminiscent of the T.V. series: Dr. Ben Casey. At times we had to contend with general surgeons regarding O.R. priority. Dr. Ruth Jacoby, the *first* Board-certified female neurosurgeon in the United States served as our chief. During the following year (as Chief Resident at the University Hospital) I acted as first assistant to Dr. Watts and other senior private neurosurgeons. My 7th year following graduation from medical school (1966-7) was truly an enjoyable, rewarding experience which included 6 months at the D.C. Children's hospital followed by 6 months at the new Veteran's Administration facility where I performed at least 80% of the surgery.

In July 1967, as an officer of the USAF, I was assigned as one of two staff neurosurgeons to the 400 bed hospital, Keesler AFB, Biloxi, Miss. In this facility we treated patients (including newborns with spina bifida}, young airmen and families (some retired) from all over the Southeast USA. During my two years as a USAF neurosurgeon I had only 4 postoperative deaths including one brain tumor and one cerebral aneurysm. In addition two patients died following traumatic paralyzing spinal injuries. I am not aware of any of my patients harboring brain or spine infections. One can only maintain the highest regard for the dedicated nursing personnel who supported our patients. While it is true that we were not treating soldiers brought from filthy trenches, muddy battlefields or enemy prisons, clearly there is ample evidence to suggest that by 1967 Medicine had indeed emerged "from the Dark Ages".

Chapter 14

Challenge of Protozoan and Fungal illness in mid twentieth century

Progress in medical and surgical therapy in addition to public health during the century following the American Civil War generally dwarfs advances in these areas achieved during the previous millennia in Western Civilization. No longer must women fear life-threatening post-partum infection transmitted by unwashed practitioners as in the days of Semmelweiss in Vienna. Individuals with wounds (accidental or surgical) of the extremities rarely experience amputation. Tuberculosis, where it still exists, is largely manageable by antibiotic therapy while many infectious illnesses can be prevented by immunization.

However in spite of intense efforts certain major disabling and life-threatening diseases remain uncontrolled. Colonization of large parts of the world, particularly in tropical areas, has enhanced spread and limited our ability to eradicate certain conditions prevalent in the "third world". It is now estimated that nearly 500 million people are infected with malaria worldwide yielding about 2.5,000,000 deaths yearly.[150] Evidence accumulated in the 19th century that the disease

---

150 Koprowski, Hillary. *Microbe Hunters Then and Now*. Bloomington, Ill :Medi-Press,1996, p367.

was caused by plasmodia and spread by mosquitoes. Finallly in 1880 Dr. Laveran, working in Algeria, identified plasmodium oocysts by carefully dissecting the stomach wall of Anopheles mosquitoes. At last the missing link between mosquito vector and human beings was revealed. At first DDT proved effective but mosquitoes rapidly developed resistance. Chloroquine was useful in treating individuals already infected but the plasmodium parasite soon became resistant to both quinine and chloroquine By the end of the 20th century malaria was believed to have caused deaths of one million children in Sub-Saharan Africa.

A second devastating illness, endemic in Africa, recognized as early as the 14th century by explorers is "sleeping sickness" resulting from infection by trypanosomes. The illness is reported to have devastated whole villages in the 19th century. Colonization promoted by Stanley (explorer) at the behest of King Leopold of Belgium was believed to have pushed the disease into the Central Congo. Extensive studies were undertaken first at the London School of Tropical Medicine by Dr. Castellani. Further studies at the Liverpool School of Tropical Medicine near the turn of the century identified trypanosomes in the blood of a shipmaster suffering from "Gambia fever".[151] In 1903 Castellani and Major David Bruce found trypanosomes in the cerebrospinal fluid of patients still alive with "sleeping sickness".[152]. In the 21st century several drugs have been found effective in control of this disease including Pentamidine and Nigurtimax.

Whereas management of wound infection and systemic infectious disease caused by bacteria and viruses has repeatedly been explored in this volume, little attention has been given to illness attributable to fungi. While not nearly as common as most other infectious processes, coccidioidomycosis was first identified during the last

---

[151] Porter, Roy. The Greatest Benefit to Mankind. New York, London: Horton and Company, 1997, p478.

[152] Porter, Roy. The Greatest Benefit to Mankind. New York, London: Horton and Company, 1997, pp477-478.

decade of the nineteenth century. Due to its prevalence in California's San Joaquin valley it came to be known as "Valley Fever". Inhalation of fungal spores commonly results in pulmonary infection often misdiagnosed as community acquired pneumonia. While there is no vaccine available, the disease can be treated with Amphotericin B which first became available in 1956. While Coccidioidomycosis is endemic in California it is also prevalent in Arizona, Nevada and New Mexico. Individuals infected with HIV are especially susceptible compared to the average person.

Histoplasmosis is a fungal infection endemic in certain areas of North and South America as well as Africa and Asia. Most cases in the U.S. have been found in the Ohio and Mississippi valleys. Although many patients do not require formal treatment, "certain forms of Histoplasmosis cause life-threatening illness and result in considerable mortality".[153] Treatment with Amphotericin-B is indicated for acute diffuse pulmonary infection and disseminated infection especially when it involves the central nervous system.[154] Additional agents which can be administered by mouth are Ketoconazole and Itraconazole. No treatment of value was available until the mid–twentieth century. Several additional fungal infections have been recognized including Blastomycosis, Cryptococcosis, and Candidiasis which can be treated with the same antifungal medications. Unfortunately the fungi have no susceptibility to bacterial antibiotics.

---

153 Wheat, L. Joseph, Freifeld, Alison G., Kleiman Martin B. et al. "Clinical Practice Guidelines for the Management of Patients with Histoplasmosis" *2007 Update.* CID 2007:45.

154 Wheat, L. Joseph, Freifeld, Alison G., Kleiman Martin B. et al. "Clinical Practice Guidelines for the Management of Patients with Histoplasmosis". *2007 Update.* CID 2007:45

Chapter 15

Nutritional essentials: The role of selectivity in health and disease

As has been suggested in an earlier chapter, physicians, nurses, and members of the Sanitary Commission recognized the general importance of the role played by adequate nutrition in recovery of soldiers from wounds and disease during the American Civil War. However identification of specific required dietary components had not been accomplished prior to the late 19th century. Scurvy among sailors of the Royal Navy had been successfully treated by providing fresh citrus fruit (such as limes)in the diet but identification of the active compound (vitamin C) was delayed until the 20th century. Normal wound healing does *not* occur in the vitamin C deficient individual.[155]

A condition known as beriberi was recognized in the rice cultures of Asia. Poorly understood, it was manifested by weakness and numbness of the extremities and later cardiac failure.[156] In 1872, 25 sailors succumbed to this malady during a long cruise on a Japanese

---

[155] Porter, Roy. *The Greatest Benefit to Mankind*. New York, London: Horton and Company, 1997, pp 555-556.

[156] Porter, Roy. *The Greatest Benefit to Mankind*. New York, London: Horton and Company, 1997, pp553-554.

naval vessel. Finally in 1912 a Polish biochemist, Casimir Funk, found that birds fed on polished rice developed a disease which resembled beriberi. He showed that marked neuromuscular weakness especially in the legs could be reversed by feeding patients whole grain rice. Funk named the critical substance contained in unpolished rice vitamin B1 (Thiamin). Shortly thereafter a second nutritional disorder whose symptoms included diarrhea, dermatitis and dementia was identified: Pellagra. This syndrome was especially prevalent in the American South where "fatback" pork containing little protein was widely consumed. Pellagra was subsequently confirmed as a deficiency in vitamin B2.[157]

Although Funk had shown that Scurvy was due to deficiency of vitamin C in the early 1900's, the substance was not isolated until 1928 by Szent –Gyorgyi. It was finally synthesized in 1932 as hexuronic acid. During the 1930's and 1940's vitamins E, G, H, and K were synthesized. During this period, following research by Dr. Whipple, Minot and Murphy showed that one form of anemia (failure of the body to make red blood cells) was related to lack of a substance later named B12 *(extrinsic* factor). It was found that certain individuals lacked a compound *(intrinsic* factor) secreted by the stomach which allowed absorption of B12 from food. In 1925 these workers showed that the anemia could be corrected by feeding the patients large quantities of liver. Following its isolation, B12 could be administered by injection. More recent studies indicated that lack of *intrinsic* factor was due to autoimmune destruction of lining cells of the stomach.

---

[157] Porter, Roy. *The Greatest Benefit to Mankind*. New York, London: Horton and Company, 1997, p554.

Chapter 16

Part 1: Poisoning: Intentional and accidental

The role of chemical and biological toxins in human health has been recognized since ancient times. Socrates was forced to ingest Hemlock with resultant death. Shakespeare described the poisoning of Hamlet's father although we are unaware of the chemical nature of this substance. The deadly effects of snake venom have been observed for centuries. Advances in organic chemistry and pharmacology have allowed analysis of the mechanism of poisoning by plant derivatives such as belladonna (atropine) and ergot (rye fungus}. Modern technology allowed mass production of poisonous inhalants during WWI including Chlorine and mustard gas. By mid-twentieth century organic-phosphate nerve agents such as DFP and later Sarin appeared. Undoubtedly the largest number of *intentional* deaths by poisoning can be attributed to the use of hydrogen cyanide in the Nazi concentration camps during WWII.

During the twentieth century treatment for arsenic and mercury poisoning was developed utilizing Dimercaprol (BAL) which prevents the binding of these metals to body cells. Lead poisoning due to chewing of peeling lead-based paint produced a serious threat to children Modern supportive care includes careful monitoring and adjustment of blood electrolytes, a tool not readily available until the 1930's. Additionally leaching of lead compounds into the water supply from outdated pipes has occurred in a number of cities. Prolonged exposure to lead impairs bone marrow, liver, kidney and brain function, but can now be treated with the chelating agent (DMSA (succimer). A second drug EDTA is available for acute life-threatening lead intoxication. Antidotes have also been developed for two of the deadliest substances known to man. Cyanide compounds which block all intracellular metabolism can be neutralized by urgent treatment with sodium thiosulfate while "nerve agents" such as Sarin can be detached by administration of pralidoxime (PAM).

Chapter 16

Part 2: Opioid crisis

In 1839 the imperial Chinese commissioner ordered foreign traders to surrender their opium. The subsequent "Opium Wars" fought by the British against China appear to have heralded the modern use of medicinal compounds for recreational purposes by a society. Essentially, the British government having succeeded in addicting a sufficient portion of the Chinese population to the use of opium, determined to ensure continued importation of this dangerous drug by force. The exchange of opium for silver proved to be the main motivating force in this enterprise. Adrian Bonenberger suggests that introduction of the hypodermic syringe around the era of the American Civil War contributed to post-war *addiction* of veterans. Synthesis of diacetyl morphine led to the distribution of the drug as "heroin" in 1898 according to Roy Porter.

The technologically advanced society which exists today-especially in the United States-has produced an almost insatiable demand for therapeutic intervention by physicians. In an earlier section I described the very limited therapeutic options available to physicians prior to WWII. In order to fulfill society's demands from a medical standpoint innumerable "patent" medicines were produced by manufacturers small and large. Prior to WWI there was essentially no effort to regulate these products almost all of which contained substances of no therapeutic value. Most commonly the contents of these "over the counter "concoctions were dissolved in solutions consisting of (ethyl) alcohol and/or opiates. Not surprisingly consumers often felt improved after ingestion. At the beginning of the twentieth century preparations containing narcotics were sold by drugstores and mail order houses without prescription. Apparently the significance of drug addiction was identified in the Philippines during the Spanish-American War leading to an International Conference called for by Theodore Roosevelt. The president appointed Dr. Hamilton Wright as the first Opium Commissioner of the United States in 1908. In 1911 Dr. Wright was noted by the New York Times to have reported that the United States consumes the most habit-forming drugs per capita of all the nations in the world." The Pure Food and Drug Act of 1906 required labeling of patent medicines which contained opiates, cocaine, alcohol and cannabis." It was estimated that one citizen in four hundred was addicted to some form of opium.

In 1914 Congress passed the Harrison Narcotics Act which amounted essentially to a tax on opium for purposes of government revenue. Charges for violations were restricted to dishonest reporting and record keeping. Dispensing was *not* a criminal offense. In 1916 the question of who could control narcotics distribution was brought before the Supreme Court. The case was dismissed on grounds that distribution of medicine was regulated under States Rights. In 1919 the Supreme Court ruled that physicians could not prescribe narcotics for maintenance of addicts. Additional Federal control of addictive substances was introduced by passage of the 18th Amendment which prohibited the sale and distribution of alcoholic beverages. A government Narcotics division was developed, headed by Levi G. Nutt, around 1920. Hundreds of pounds of opium and morphine were seized resulting in 1583 convictions in 1921. The Jones-Miller Act of 1922 prohibited importation of opium for other than medicinal purposes. Certain individuals believed that addicts were principal incubators of streptococcus, pneumococcus, influenza and tuberculosis. In 1930 the FBN (Federal Bureau of Narcotics) was established under president Hoover. Interdiction of international drug trade led to seizure of 150 pounds of heroin from the French liner Ile de France. From a cargo marked "furs" agents recovered 1000 pounds of morphine hidden on the cargo ship Alesia enroute from Istanbul to Brooklyn. Reduction in supply of illegal narcotics found addicts searching for bottles of Paregoric(an anti-diarrheal) from which opium could be extracted. Participation in the illegal drug trade led to arrest of various Mafia members.

Following WWII the FBN was given jurisdiction over newly developed synthetic painkillers such as Demerol and Dilaudid. The Boggs-Daniel Narcotics control Act of 1956 raised the minimum sentence for first offense narcotics trafficking to 5 years in prison increasing to10-40 years for subsequent conviction. All heroin was ordered to be removed from shelves within 120 days. Subsequently the New York Mafia boss Vito Genovese was convicted and sent to prison where he died of natural causes. In 1960 Mauricio Rosal, Guatemalan Ambassador to the Netherlands, was sentenced to 15 years in prison for illegal drug trafficking after 100 pounds of heroin was unpacked from his luggage.

In addition to drug–related crime the proliferation of "Street Drug" usage has resulted in an ever increasing mortality from drug overdose particularly in individuals between 15 and 35. A new organization: the DEA was created in 1973 to closely monitor narcotics prescriptions which were believed to trigger addiction in many individuals. Often when prescriptions can no longer be legitimately obtained, dependency drives users to buy narcotics illegally-the strength or potency of which is unknown even to sellers. The death toll in the USA from overdose has climbed from 19,000 in 1999 to over 65,000 in 2016. Although poisoning and death from drugs remains a "new Dark Age" in Medicine, it is encouraging to note that the growth rate in death from *prescription* opioids has decreased from 13% to 4.8%. Although Nalline (Nalorphine) was described in my medical school pharmacology course in 1957, Naloxone has only recently been released to the public as a lifesaving opioid antidote.

Endnotes

In this brief discussion of recent medical history I have tried to enable the reader to appreciate the dramatic improvement in health care delivery which occurred during the century following the American Civil War. In reference one might compare the efficiency of trans-Atlantic transport by sail to that of ocean-going steamships during the last quarter of the 19th century.

All too frequently one is tempted to believe that accurate diagnostic information and successful management of illness has been available for an indefinite period of time. One need only reflect on the deficiencies described in this volume which persisted well into the 20th century to appreciate the remarkably rapid evolution of medical care which we regularly enjoy today.

END

www.ingramcontent.com/pod-product-compliance
Lightning Source LLC
Chambersburg PA
CBHW020446220526
45464CB00002B/876